HIV and Learning Disability

British Library Cataloguing in Publication Data

A CIP record for this book is available from the British Library

ISBN 1 873791 91 7

Copyright © 1997 **bild** Publications

bild Publications is the publishing office of the
British Institute of Learning Disabilities
Wolverhampton Road
Kidderminster
Worcestershire
United Kingdom DY10 3PP
telephone 01562 850251
fax 01562 851970
e-mail bild@bild.demon.co.uk.

bild Publications are distributed worldwide by
Plymbridge Distributors Limited
Estover House
Plymouth
United Kingdom PL6 7PZ
telephone 01752 202300
fax 01752 202333.

Printed by The Cookley Printers Limited
56 Bridge Road
Cookley
Kidderminster
Worcestershire
United Kingdom DY10 3SB.

CONTENTS

i

INTRODUCTION

Paul Cambridge writes.

The aim of this book is to provide essential reference material for people working in the field of HIV and learning disability. For this reason it has a clear practice bias, drawing on the experience of successful services and practitioners already working in the field in innovative ways. Best practice does not exist in a vacuum however; therefore some chapters include analyses of relevant management and organisation issues. By providing an assessment of competence in responding to HIV in learning disability the book should help people respond more effectively, not only to the challenge of HIV but also to sexuality more widely. For instance, safer sex education should be an integral part of work in sexuality and sex education and address issues of power, control, exploitation and abuse.

HIV has caused terrible suffering and anguish to those affected directly and indirectly. Like many other gay men and many other people without a gay or lesbian identity, I think of my friends who have died from AIDS and those who have lost their friends or the people they loved and enjoyed life with. Sometimes ordinary events, comments or places can evoke vivid images which are almost impossible to bear. There are millions of similar thoughts and experiences on every continent at any one time. AIDS is not something any of us can turn away from and we have to live with it and fight it individually and collectively. By pooling our diverse experiences, knowledge and skills we can regain some control over something of which we still have no idea where it is leading us.

Rather than a global pandemic, there are different epidemics, affecting different groups of people, for different reasons, in different parts of the world. In Britain, it is mainly men who have sex with men who have been most affected. In other parts of the world, economically or socially disadvantaged groups are disproportionately affected by HIV. The global melting pot is blurring the edges of the different epidemics and has given rise to some of the "most unacceptable" characteristics of human nature, including racism, homophobia, blame and victimisation. In North America and Western Europe, gay men have successfully *re-gayed* AIDS and have fought back through direct action and self help, using buddy services, safer sex campaigns and direct action against homophobia. This struggle is necessarily political and unfortunately people with learning disabilities lack the power and organisations to fight back because of social and economic constraints.

Fortunately, many gay men have used their experiences of HIV and sexuality to inform work in the learning disability community, in the same ways as others have brought their values and commitment to fighting prejudice to their own work in HIV and AIDS. Learning disability services continue to be largely exclusive of gay spaces, although men with learning disabilities may access spaces where gay men and others who have sex with men meet. It is perhaps no coincidence that both learning disability and gay spaces are policed informally and formally in relation to sexuality and men with learning disabilities encounter big disadvantages in their sexual encounters with other men with or without learning disabilities.

Few good things come out of our experience of HIV and AIDS, but one has been to bring sexuality out of the closet and to break down some of the societal barriers to honesty and openness about sexual behaviour and sexual feelings. The choice is stark. We develop a radical discourse and effective interventions in our work in HIV and learning disability or we perpetuate myth and ignorance and the disadvantage and inequalities they bring. The fight against AIDS is also a fight for our rights as individuals and communities. This experience can be positively used to empower people with learning disabilities to recognise their rights to sexual expression and relationships and to safety from abuse, exploitation and HIV.

We both write....

Chapter 1 argues for the re-homosexualisation of HIV and AIDS in services for people with learning disabilities. It identifies the structural and organisational factors which determine how needs are recognised and services and resources in HIV and learning disability are commissioned. The needs of men with learning disabilities who have sex with men are urgent in relation to HIV, because unlike *gay identified* men they do not have access to peer education and support and are less aware of the HIV risks attached to their sexual encounters.

In Chapter 2, Jan Welch provides an explanation of HIV infection and AIDS in terms of transmission, virology and treatment. Our understanding of HIV and AIDS has increased dramatically over the last decade, but although we have developed medical interventions to effectively treat many AIDS related illnesses, there is no vaccine or cure. It is important that we have an accurate but straightforward idea of how HIV is transmitted, how HIV infection develops into AIDS and what to expect in relation to illness and treatment if we are to respond with appropriate information and support to someone with a learning disability.

The key role health promotion services can play in pump priming and co-ordinating local initiatives in relation to HIV and learning disability is demonstrated by James Nichol in Chapter 3. From a review of health promotion models, a strong case is made for multi-agency working to develop an approach to sexual health which is grounded in the reality of risk and operationalised through radical and effective service models.

In Chapter 4, Simon Davies describes work with one young man in a residential service who is at high risk of HIV infection. The importance of constructing valued and enabling social environments is demonstrated, along with the resource implications for service providers and managers. There are considerations for staff culture, including attitudes, support space, dignity and respect. Services for people with learning disabilities need to plan but also to respond in unique ways, developing skills in risk assessment and risk management.

David Thompson explains in Chapter 5 how men with learning disabilities are socialised not to talk about sex with men. This presents a special challenge to sex educators in their work to combat the denial of same sex relationships, as it is one of the main disincentives to practising safer sex. Help with developing a positive self image and the assertiveness needed to negotiate safer sex is therefore required in same sex encounters as it is for women in their encounters with men.

In Chapter 6, Michelle McCarthy identifies a range of possible priorities for individual and group sex education, stressing the role of the educator as information giver. Her work with women indicates the need to empower women to negotiate safer sex and to be more assertive in saying no to sex that they do not enjoy. Experience suggests that simply providing condoms in no way equates with their effective use. The barrier between knowledge and behaviour is one sex educators need to help dismantle.

The potential role for therapeutic interventions as a route to help combat the negative consequences of abusive or unsafe sexual experiences are explained by Stephen Morris in Chapter 7. People with learning disabilities pick up negative messages from various sources about their learning disability and how society devalues them and such images need to be overcome before they can be empowered to practice safer sex. To many people with learning disabilities the threat to life from AIDS is just one more threat to their existence.

In Chapter 8 Fiona Barber and Paul Redfern demonstrate that people with learning disabilities can themselves be empowered to make sexual choices and helped to understand HIV and AIDS through self advocacy and peer education. Their observations stress the importance of constructing and using visual images to help people, who may have limited literacy skills, to exercise choice in safer sex and other aspects of personal and sexual relationships.

David Sewart relates the problems and potentials of providing sex and safer sex education for young people with learning disabilities in Chapter 9. His work clearly points to the gains and benefits of pro-activity in curriculum development and work with parents and other interest groups.

In his review of HIV and the law in learning disability in Chapter 10, Michael Gunn explains the potential pressures on services to properly manage HIV risk and related issues such as informed consent for HIV testing. The responsibilities that services have for providing competent support for people at risk of HIV or with HIV or AIDS and their wider responsibilities for protecting service users and others from the risk of HIV are explained in ordinary language.

Policies and procedures are needed to develop competence for working with people with learning disabilities on sexuality and HIV and Chapter 11 provides a framework and pointers for a way forward. We stress the vital role policies and guidelines can play for management and practice and how they help to co-ordinate action and clarify responsibility and accountability.

Hilary Brown writes...

It is usual in jointly edited books to co-write an introduction which sets out a shared view of the material to follow and shared reference points against which editorial decisions have been made. In this instance however, we felt it more appropriate to write separately about our journey to these issues and commitment to them and to identify the distinct editorial approaches we have applied to the book. We hope we have complemented each other.

In his introductory comments, Paul Cambridge writes from his experience as a gay man. His commitment to people with learning disabilities in relation to HIV issues grows out of a wider political experience; seeking to extend the solidarity and honesty with which gay men and their organisations, have tackled issues of HIV prevention and support to each other and to people with learning disabilities.

My own experience as a straight woman has been in recognising and co-ordinating responses to the sexual abuse and exploitation of people with learning disabilities; an area which has not been explicitly acknowledged until relatively recently. The nature of sexual abuse revealed in recent surveys (Brown, Stein & Turk, 1995; McCarthy & Thompson forthcoming), forces us to find words to speak of people's vulnerability, as well as their rights to and rights in, sexual encounters. The continued devaluation of people with learning disabilities within the wider community, their lack of knowledge and support, the equivocal respect accorded to their credibility, make them vulnerable in their sexual encounters. Meanwhile, within the confines of service cultures and spaces, a strict hierarchy operates wherein gender, power and ability intersect to produce, too often, relationships and acts marked by and based on inequality and coercion rather than mutuality and consent.

Moreover we see that sexualities are forged in relation to economic and social realities and in the case of people with learning disabilities grow out of their marginalisation and lack of resources or personal options. The truth is that men with learning disabilities are not a powerful group even when they compensate by exploiting each other or women with learning disabilities.

Despite tremendous strides in the last two decades the response of services to the personal and sexual disadvantages of individuals with learning disabilities remains tenuous. A false dichotomy is often set up whereby services characterise their stance as primarily one of protection *or* empowerment, as if the two were in opposition. The result is that services, which seek to 'allow' people to enjoy sexual options, frequently operate in a laissez-faire mode, thereby avoiding contentious issues or explicit advocacy and support, whereas services which operate in a protective mode close off positive options.

And yet, as Paul Cambridge and many of the writers of chapters in this book demonstrate, good practice in this area demands clarity and the courage of explicit convictions. If the civil liberties of people with learning disabilities are to be restored and maintained, their rights to the sex they seek and to protection from sex which they do not want, or cannot consent to, must be *actively* supported. Within this commitment an equivalent stance must be taken on behalf of men with learning disabilities who want and have sex with men. Dilution or rejection of this experience as legitimate works against their interests when it comes to safer sex education, counselling and advocacy.

Until and unless rights to same sex relationships are guaranteed and those relationships valued and made visible in services for people with learning disabilities, individuals are at double jeopardy in their sexual lives. They remain unsafe and unsupported in the very services which exist to act on their behalf. This is a potentially fatal situation for the people themselves and represents a stance which borders on negligence on the part of service agencies. It is an abdication of responsibility which all those concerned in the provision of services must counter.

Chapter 1

Assessing and Responding to Local Needs in HIV and Learning Disability

by Paul Cambridge

Commissioners have the duty to specify and purchase a comprehensive range of local services designed to meet the needs of the populations they serve. This chapter looks at the level of competence in needs assessment and commissioning in HIV and learning disability and the value and appropriateness of different resources and specialist services. Evidence on the location and nature of need is examined in relation to men with learning disabilities who have sex with men and the best ways to meet needs are discussed. The context of the care market and the structural and organisational disincentives to effective service planning and development are also considered. Pointers for best practice in developing safer sex, educational resources, and HIV risk assessment and risk management skills are suggested, with an overview of the service options in HIV and learning disability.

The Evidence

The epidemiology of HIV infection in Britain has been characterised by as much myth as has AIDS itself. The *gaying* of AIDS in the early years of the epidemic was represented by the scapegoating of gay men and further pathologising of homosexuality, with variations of *gay plague* headlines and articles in the popular press. The *de-gaying* of AIDS in the late 1980s was partly a response to this irrational homophobia but also to the fear that HIV would cross into the general (heterosexual) population, with AIDS developing into a more widespread epidemic. It was exemplified by health promotion campaigns and Government television advertising aimed primarily at preventing heterosexual transmission, promoting safer sex and discouraging casual sex. The *re-gaying* of AIDS in the 1990s was a political response by organised gay men to the reality of where HIV risk and AIDS related needs continued to be located in the population, namely with gay men and other men who have sex with men. By this time other high risk groups were also evident, such haemophiliacs who had received infected blood products and people who shared needles for intravenous drug use, but gay men remained most affected.

The *re-gaying* of AIDS helped a reappraisal of how HIV prevention work could be most productively targeted and where health and social care services were required. It helped to bring gay led organisations like Gay Men Fighting AIDS (founded in 1992) more prominently into campaigning against homophobia, promoting safer sex and monitoring the provision of specialist services. This shift helped to compensate for over a decade of neglect, as King (1993) has observed:

'With the benefit of hindsight ... one can only conclude that the dehomosexualisation of AIDS has led directly to the marginalisation of gay men's unparalleled experience and contributions to fighting the epidemic, and has ultimately exacerbated the harmful effects of the epidemic on those who are most at risk'. (p.170).

This reappraisal of HIV risk and need, driven by the reality of experience, also has implications for HIV prevention work in learning disability. The arguments presented in this chapter are based on the hypothesis that sex education and HIV prevention resources for people with learning disabilities have failed to respond effectively to HIV risk and that there are areas where HIV prevention work in services for people with learning disabilities could productively learn from the experience of sexual health promotion for and by gay men. In effect, I will argue for the re-homosexualisation of HIV and AIDS in services for people with learning disabilities. But in making these arguments I do not intend to distract attention from the risk of HIV to women with learning disabilities or fail to acknowledge their particular sexual experiences (McCarthy, 1994 - see also Chapter 6).

Men who have sex with men continue to be disproportionately represented in the UK statistics from voluntary named testing for known HIV infection and reported AIDS cases.

'By the end of 1993, there had been a cumulative total of 13,015 men with HI V-1 infection acquired via sex with other men, 62% of total infections reported since 1984... AIDS cases amongst gay and bisexual men comprised 78% of all the adult AIDS cases reported since the start of the epidemic, and 70% of adult cases reported from January to December 1993' (Rooney, 1994, p.53).

Despite overpowering evidence of where need lies in relation to HIV and AIDS in the UK population (the over-representation of gay and bisexual men in the HIV and AIDS statistics represents a hugely disproportionate impact on minority communities), the *de-gaying* of AIDS led to HIV prevention resources being poorly targeted and therefore ineffectively used. This argument is powerfully articulated by King (1993) who observed only three years ago that out of the fifteen or more posts in HIV or AIDS that the Health Education Authority had established, only one was specifically for men who have sex with men, with evidence of budget reductions in HEA funding for campaigns targeting gay men and that these campaigns represented under 20% of the overall AIDS budget (Pink Paper, 1992). The mis-targeting of HIV prevention resources and initiatives is echoed by others involved in HIV prevention activities

'It is dismaying that two thirds of the agencies surveyed reported that they were not engaged in any kind of HIV prevention work targeting gay or bisexual men' (King, Rooney & Scott, 1992, p.23).

It is important to acknowledge the diversity of sexual behaviours found in any community of interest or identity, be it lesbian, bisexual, gay or people with learning disabilities. This is necessary in order to appreciate the complexities of HIV prevention work. While the aggregate statistical evidence points to gay men and other men who have sex with men as a high HIV risk group, there is also evidence to suggest a diversity of sexual behaviours, lifestyles and responses to HIV risk within this population. More importantly, while there is evidence to support the assumption that safer sex interventions work in reducing HIV infection (Berkelman et al, 1989), wider data suggests that an increase in knowledge about safer sex is not necessarily associated with the practice of safer sex (Davies et al, 1993). Project SIGMA (Social-sexual Investigation of Gay Men and AIDS) tracked a cohort of more than 1,000 men over a four year period to examine their social and sexual behavioural responses to HIV. It revealed a high level of knowledge about safer sex but variable responses to HIV risk. Previous research into homosexual behaviour had also suggested a similar variety in relationships, numbers of sexual partners and sexual identities (Kinsey, 1948). Needs assessment work, HIV prevention campaigns and direct safer sex education should therefore recognise and respond to this diversity, including work in learning disability.

No service for people with learning disabilities or any service commissioner is immune from HIV as a management or practice issue. The evidence from sex education (McCarthy & Thompson, 1994), peer education (People First, 1994), counselling and therapeutic services (Morris, 1993), sexual health outreach (Jones, 1993) and research (Cambridge, 1996a) indicates significant levels of risk or case examples of high risk sexual activities and the imperative to develop appropriate HIV prevention responses. More widely, little is known about the epidemiology of HIV infection in people with learning disabilities (Simonds & Rogers, 1992), although it is known that people with learning disabilities have become infected with HIV (Kastner et al, 1992; 1989). As with other individuals and populations, the nature and level of risk varies: the person with profound learning disabilities who cannot communicate verbally and who is sexually abused; the man with learning disabilities who frequently has unsafe sex with anonymous partners in public toilets; the woman with learning disabilities who sometimes has sex for money or cigarettes; and the young person with learning disabilities developing their first sexual feelings or relying on intimate care. All have different needs for education and protection. Segregation in services is not the same thing as isolation from the wider community and provides no protection against HIV.

Assessing Need

In recognition of the political and moral imperative behind the re-gaying of AIDS, South East London Health Authority funded research and training for men with learning disabilities who have sex with men in public places, putting the question firmly on the commissioning agenda (Cambridge et al, 1994). The needs assessment component of the project indicated that a number of men with learning disabilities in SE London were at high risk of HIV infection and that some services had difficulties responding to this risk (Cambridge, 1994). This alerted commissioners to the risks of not responding to the needs of this group of men, although evidence from sex education (Thompson D, 1994) and needs assessment in mainstream sexual health (Taylor-Laybourn & Aggleton, 1992) also indicated that some men with learning disabilities were at high risk of HIV.

There are many potential explanations as to why men with learning disabilities are likely to be vulnerable to HIV risk from having sex in public places and these are summarised in Box 1. They include both individual and environmental considerations and some can be influenced by the power of the support services.

Box I
VULNERABILITY TO HIV

histories of institutionalisation, social de-skilling and the development of acquiescence and dependency in congregate settings

community services find normalisation and community integration difficult principles to practice, and this is reflected in difficulties supporting sexuality

poor sex and safer sex education, lack of access to condoms, little assertiveness training and poor negotiation skills for safer sex

poor staff training, low competence to recognise and respond to HIV; need and lack of policies and guidelines on sexuality

secrecy and guilt about sexualities; pathological view of homosexuality and disincentives to identify as gay

emotional vulnerability and desire to seek out friendships and social contacts; easy targets for intimidation and control and hence abuse and exploitation

lack of privacy, confidentiality, dignity and respect in residential and other support services

little politicisation, self organisation and peer support, with isolation in services

invisibility of homosexual role models; lack of opportunities to choose sexual options and low economic status to facilitate participation.

SELHA was responsible for funding both learning disability services and HIV/AIDS services and had earmarked resources for HIV prevention and health promotion (the context is explained by James Nichol in Chapter 3). The results highlighted important considerations for commissioners and providers on the needs of the high HIV risk group of men who have sex with men, with a focus on men with learning disabilities who go cottaging (have sex in public toilets). These are summarised below (see Cambridge, 1996a for a more detailed report)

- there was a significant prevalence of men with learning disabilities known *and* reported to be possibly or definitely cottaging (the total in Lewisham, Lambeth and Southwark was 34). This is likely to be an under-estimate considering the problems associated with the

5

recognition and reporting of similar issues such as sexual abuse
(Brown et al., 1995). Many men in this situation hide their behaviour
because they think it is wrong or because it contradicts their social and
sexual identity (Thompson, 1994).

- men with learning disabilities who have sex with men in public toilets
  are at an especially high risk of HIV. Rarely are they in a position to
  insist on or practice safer sex, they have different sexual partners and
  they are usually penetrated anally or orally by men from a high risk
  group. One service responded *'he visits the local cottage up to seven
  times a week and has regular unprotected anal intercourse'*, and another
  observed *'the client meets men in public toilets and goes back to their
  homes with them'*.

- the median age of the men in the sample was 30, and 80% had good
  communication skills. They were therefore a relatively young and able
  group of men, although they were supported by a wide range of
  residential services, including hospitals, hostels, group homes and
  unstaffed housing, therefore need is clearly spread across the range of
  formal support services. A number of indicators of risk were identified
  and these included the obvious: a history of STD or being escorted
  home by the police and the less obvious: regular absence from services
  and reluctance to say where they had been.

- over 40% of the men in the sample definitely had sex with other men
  with learning disabilities and over 21% definitely had sex with women
  with learning disabilities. This raises critical questions for managing
  HIV risk within services. For example *'he has a steady girlfriend and
  several other women friends with whom he may also be having sex'*.
  Service users have freedoms and rights as well as responsibilities in
  relation to minimising HIV risks to sexual partners. This raises
  conflicting service responsibilities for protecting people from an
  unacceptable risk of HIV, while promoting and safeguarding rights and
  respecting privacy and confidentiality.

- risk assessment and risk management skills were poorly developed,
  although this in part reflected the skills of men in hiding their
  behaviours and their reluctance to talk with staff about what they did.
  Most providers did not hold a refined understanding of HIV or safer sex

or the competence to provide educational inputs, for instance one service responded that a man they supported '*was advised to use condoms and given a supply but does not like using them and gives inconsistent replies*' and another that '*the staff team can only speculate at this moment in time. If he is cottaging, then we don't know if he is practising safer sex.*'

HIV and learning disability is an area where joint commissioning offers considerable potential. There is currently an implementation gap in commissioning and providing learning disability services competent at working in HIV and HIV and AIDS services, such as genito-urinary medicine (GUM) clinics, competent at working with people with learning disabilities. Some specialist services bridge the gap, but most people with learning disabilities fail to get support for managing informed consent for sex, assertiveness for determining sex and using condoms, providing condoms, assessing valid consent for HIV testing and access to pre - and post - test counselling. Approaches to HIV testing can indicate levels of competence in the management and practice of HIV and is revisited later in the chapter.

Managing the Market

Consideration needs to be given to the market in social and community care (the separation of purchasing and providing and the contract), when assessing how to recognise, respond and *most effectively* meet needs in HIV and learning disability. This is because needs are largely met through market formulated responses, and effective service development in HIV and learning disability will require an assessment of local market conditions. The market, as it has been operating and developing since the 1990 health and community care reforms, has demanded increasing management skills (HMSO, 1992; DoH, 1993). Processes such as joint commissioning, community care planning and care management and the contract itself can be used to help manage the market more pro-actively and assertively. For instance, commissioning can be used to specify radical service models, such as sex education or counselling services, within a coherent philosophy and local strategy. Individual contracts can be used to specify requirements for group or individual sex education or HIV risk management and involve people in determining their own services (Brown & Cambridge, 1995).

Commissioners should give preference to those arrangements they believe, or there is evidence to suggest, generate the most productive outcomes in the lives of the people who use services. There is little objective evidence about such associations in sexual health and learning disability and there has been limited experience or time to develop radical models. Pilot demonstration services, properly evaluated for effectiveness, are needed to better inform commissioning, although there have been isolated examples (Cambridge, 1996b). Some of the accounts in following chapters represent an informal approach to posing and answering related questions about the effectiveness and values of model services. Commissioners do not live in a different political or social world to others. They are as open to ignorance and bigotry about HIV and AIDS and to homophobia as anyone else, although the political context to commissioning is significant, as the SE London work illustrates, and it is on such information that services should be developed.

The people who use learning disability services cannot be compared with consumers in most other markets (they are more like *customers* travelling with a warrant on a partly privatised railway system). To think of people with learning disabilities as consumers with resources and choices is fantastic, other than for the few people in advocacy or service brokerage schemes. What has increasingly happened over the last five years, is that the people who use services have at best been exchanged between agencies and at worst traded as commodities. Their behaviours, skills, abilities and needs, including their needs for visible things like housing and practical support for life skills and less visible things like friendships, personal relationships and sexual expression and health have been priced and marketed. Political and financial accountability has become blurred because those who provide services are further away from those who fund them and lines of management accountability have become dislocated.

It is unusual to find sexuality and HIV referenced in contracts. Most people are still unable to choose where they live, who they live with or which agency supports them, let alone who they have sex with, what type of sex they have and whether they have safer sex. The case studies and accompanying rationales provided by Simon Davies and David Stewart in their chapters demonstrate a competence which is difficult to specify through the contract, as it depends on individual values and commitment. Similarly, the innovative work described by David Thompson and Stephen Morris in their chapters is grounded in a sexual politics which can be used to inform the nature of intervention and the professional stance. It is not just the difficulty of putting best practice into words and assessing performance in meaningful ways, but also of resolving what amount to politically contentious issues through the contract, such as responsibility for managing HIV risk and paying for educational and health services. Examples of radical approaches include: the empowerment of women at risk of sexual exploitation or HIV, sex education within a feminist discourse, sexual health outreach, support for the whole person, the provision of safe space outside services and advocacy and peer education. Such models depend on a radicalism and political activism likely to frighten commissioners. Getting radical services is a structural problem to do with who holds power more widely in society and people with learning disabilities remain socially, politically and economically marginalised, as reflected in their sexual exploitation and abuse (Turk & Brown, 1993; Brown et al, 1995).

The other side of the equation is service provision and practice. The competence of providers to recognise need, take considered steps to protect people from sexual abuse and HIV, and support people to make more informed choices or take more informed risks is also limited. Moreover, there is evidence to suggest a need to intervene to modify staff attitudes to issues such as HIV testing, as the results of a study by Murray and colleagues indicates (Murray et al, 1995). Only a small minority of providers have taken the lead in this area (the initiative to manage risks and rights described by Simon Davies in Chapter 4 is a rare example). Few providers have developed sexuality policies, especially ones based on staff needs and user experiences (Cambridge & McCarthy, 1996) and are consequently not in a good position to lobby commissioners for more resources.

Recognising Need

There is a scarcity of specialist counselling, sex education and therapeutic services in sexuality and HIV for people with learning disabilities. This is especially the case for the high HIV risk and not uncommon behaviour of men with learning disabilities who have sex with men (McCarthy & Thompson, 1994). A few specialist sexuality services working specifically in HIV and learning disability and often also in sexual abuse (as we will read in Stephen Morris's chapter), have emerged but rarely from pro-active commissioning.

Respond, the service described at the end of Stephen Morris's chapter, developed from committed individuals who recognised that an important need for counselling and therapeutic interventions within a safe space remained unmet. It has to charge for its services although local commissioners have funded some limited projects, such as sexual health outreach (Cambridge,

1996b). The individuals referred are funded by their local commissioners or providing organisations, creating real resource disincentives to access such services, as a longer term commitment is usually required.

The Sex Education Team (originally funded by Herts Health Promotion Unit but now Horizon NHS - learning disability - Trust) provides sex education at no direct cost to services or users in its area, regardless of agency or sector (although staff training is charged for), but, as a consequence, is not able to reach out beyond local boundaries (see the services described by Michelle McCarthy and David Thompson in Chapters 6 and 5).

The Tizard Centre provides some clinical work as well as staff training and policy development, but however competent specialist services are, their current dispersal and location does not facilitate equity in access, or guarantee that a balance can be struck between individual contracts and longer term development funding, making planning for the future difficult. Some local initiatives have unexpectantly had their funding cut, therefore in addition to pump-priming resources, longer term funding commitments are needed for services to have an impact on what is a longer term issue requiring ongoing investment. People working in and using specialist services cannot demand integrated and co-ordinated individual service planning, as there are also organisational and professional barriers to overcome.

Part of the dilemma of gaining funding for HIV prevention activities for any group or community extends beyond the recognition of need to include the acknowledgement of outcomes which cannot be realistically assessed. An evaluation of the interventions described in this book would require elaborate longitudinal experimental designs and control groups. This would amount to an immorality by definition of the exclusion of potentially life saving interventions to people at risk of HIV infection. As Davies et al. (1993) have commented:

> 'HIV prevention programs are bedevilled by their own success. There is no praise for seroconversions that do not happen, for lives saved or communities protected. The reward for success is, rather, to be accused of scare-mongering, of demanding special treatment, of foisting a gay liberationist agenda in the guise of health promotion' (p.173).

The task of commissioners is to respond to HIV risk in learning disability by commissioning services targeted on need, despite the probability of reactionary political pressures. An equivalent task faces those charged with responsibility for developing effective HIV prevention resources.

Images in Pictures and Language

'Resources and education campaigns have been remorselessly targeted at those at least risk of contracting HIV, as if the priority of preventing an epidemic among heterosexuals had been established at the expense of halting the epidemics that are actually raging throughout the developed world' (Watney, 1993, quoted in King, 1993, p.69).

Until the early 1990s', resources available for sex education and learning disability were predominantly heterosexual and largely avoided HIV. Mirroring the *degaying* of AIDS in the late 1980s, they missed the needs of those most at risk of HIV, namely men with learning disabilities who have sex with men (Craft, 1991; Dixon, 1991), although the significance and impact of pioneering work in sexuality should not be understated, as different demands operated. More recent resources make limited reference to HIV, safer sex and homosexuality between men (McCarthy & Thompson, 1992; SELHPS, 1992) or use pictures which neutralise gender through androgynous images (LSS, 1992). A sex education video uses puppets to represent people, with sequences of personal hygiene, social skills, masturbation and penetrative anal and vaginal sex (WLHPA, 1994). Although condoms are used for the latter two sequences, the anus on the men in the homosexual sequence is shown as a seam with shadow penetration, while there is an explicit representation of a vagina and vaginal penetration in the heterosexual sequence. Critical safer sex messages, such as how to use a condom properly during anal sex, after ejaculation and when withdrawing the penis are consequently blurred for a high risk behaviour and high risk group. Although more explicit, both in its use of actors and in the directness of sexual images, an Australian video resource (FPANSW, 1993) similarly avoids close ups of penetrative anal sex between two men while happily showing details of penetrative vaginal sex. Homosexuality continues to be marginalised, despite it being central to properly targeted and effective HIV prevention work.

Explanations for this *visible* reluctance to show clear images of men having sex with men include the possibility of homophobia in that homosexual sex is seen to be of less emotional or physical value than heterosexual sex, commercial or political concerns in relation to the marketability of such resources or legal qualms about representing homosexuality or anal sex. Recent video and photographic sex educational materials produced for and by gay men (THT, 1994; Tatchell, 1994) illustrate that explicit images of men

having sex with men, hard penises and semen can be effectively represented in a safer sex educational context.

'... *safer sex is viewed as unerotic or unexciting by many people. To maximise
the impact of safer sex information it is clearly necessary to move from
communicating about sex as a biomedical issue, to a position where safer
sex is presented in explicit and erotic ways...to emphasise the erotic
potential of safer sex*' (Deverell & Rooney, 1994, p.7).

Services and educators need positive, explicit and accurate images of men
having sex with men for effective safer sex education in learning disability.
This argument extends to the use of erotic images in the context of safer sex
education for gay men. Any debate about the level of explicitness of such
materials is a distraction from the imperative of HIV prevention, although
sexual imagery produced or used outside an educational rationale is
potentially pornographic. Resources for safer sex work in learning disability
are still inhibited by societal constraints about sex and homosexuality which
do not reflect the reality and diversity of sexual experience, but there are
problems associated with using erotic images as a vehicle to deliver safer sex
education in learning disability. The message could be misread or the
educator could find the material offensive. Images need to be accurate and
culturally appropriate and what is culturally appropriate for one gay man
may not be for another gay man or other men who have sex with men who
hold a heterosexual social identity. The latter are more likely to include men
with learning disabilities who have sex with men.

Holding a positive self-image and self-worth is a necessary prerequisite to
practicing safer sex and becoming politically active and assertive.
Organisations like OUTRAGE, Gay Men Fighting AIDS, BigUp and The
Sisters of Perpetual Indulgence directly challenge homophobia and the political
and social devaluisation of homosexuality. This is in part a response to the
ways in which homosexuality has been further pathologised since AIDS by
parts of the media and some politicians. But it is no co-incidence that these
same organisations are also active in sexual health campaigns and outreach work. Social exclusion makes this option largely inaccessible for men
with learning disabilities

The potential for erotic images of men having safer sex with men extends
beyond simply drawing attention to the underlying message about safer sex
to promoting positive self images. These are required to help combat the
guilt and secrecy sometimes associated with the sexual behaviours of men

who have sex with men, including men with learning disabilities (Thompson D, 1994). There is therefore a rationale for safer sex educational materials in learning disability to use positive images where appropriate, for instance when describing consenting sex or safer sexual practices. The line between eroticism and positive image is a fine one, but it is essential that it is explored in sex education for men with learning disabilities who have sex with men. This is not to say that all images of men having sex with men need to be positive. It is important to acknowledge exploitation and abuse in a homosexual as well as heterosexual context. We know that most abusers are men who abuse men as well as women with learning disabilities. We also know that a high proportion of the men who abuse other people with learning disabilities are service users themselves (Brown et al, 1995). This reality, however unpleasant, also needs to be represented.

One of the most creative and innovative resources available for work in learning disability (a comment also echoed by staff in staff training exercises) was produced in the Netherlands for sex education with young people (Marneth, 1994), using effective combinations of photographs, line drawings and overlays.

These include pictures of both negative and positive personal contexts to sex, different sexual behaviours, erect penises, semen, condoms on penises, semen in condoms and other considerations essential for explaining consent, safer sex and HIV risk.

Similar constraints to the use of visual images have also applied to the use of language, also creating barriers to effective communication. This stopped when gay men started producing materials and information relevant to the lives and needs of gay men. A classic example of woolly language in safer sex messages is *avoid the exchange of body fluids.* In practical safer sex terms, this means *don't fuck or suck off without a condom.* Some language used in resources designed for work with people with learning disabilities has been similarly ambiguous, although good resources should encourage the educator to use peoples' own words. An example of the latter is the video on safer sex acted by people with learning disabilities (SELHPS, 1992), which used direct words and images. This contrasts markedly with the Australian video (FPANSW, 1993) which imposes professional language onto people with learning disabilities. Most of the other experience accumulated by gay men in relation to safer sex education is also transferable to some extent to work in learning disability (Box 2).

13

> **Box 2**
> **LESSONS FROM GAY MEN'S SAFER SEX EDUCATION**
> **EXPERIENCE**
>
> don't pathologise individuals or their behaviours
>
> don't impose a moral framework: work to individuals, own assumptions and agenda
>
> don't marginalise HIV as an issue in services or general day to day work with people
>
> recognise the reality of high risk groups and risk behaviours and develop risk assessment skills
>
> respond with practical support to reduce or replace risk behaviours, rather than trying to limit sexual expression
>
> reflect the realities of sexual experience through language and image
>
> encourage positive images about self and sexual preference (identity for gay men or behaviour for men who have sex with men)
>
> promote assertiveness and negotiation for safer sex within and outside relationships
>
> use HIV testing only as part of an individual strategy to manage HIV risk
>
> provide a safe and confidential environment for this work

Straight Messages About Complex Issues

The complexities surrounding the transmission and virology of HIV and the development and treatment of AIDS have always been simplified to some extent in health promotion and HIV prevention work, including safer sex work with people with learning disabilities. HIV risk activities are presented as high, medium or low and key messages about reducing the number of sexual partners or using protection for penetrative sex are presented outside co-factors which help assess risk, such as how condoms are used or the presence of other infections. This has also been the case in safer sex education in learning disability. There are sound arguments for not distinguishing between HIV and AIDS or concentrating on high risk behaviours (see David Thompson's and Michelle McCarthy's arguments in Chapters 5 and 6 David Stewart's account of sex education for young people in Chapter 9). Many people with learning disabilities who are sexually active are also relatively able however, and the importance of maintaining safer sexual behaviour could be reinforced by a more refined understanding of HIV than simply that *you could get ill and die if you have sex without a condom.*

The central question is how best to meet the needs of people with learning disabilities for information on HIV, AIDS and safer sex without excluding them from sexual opportunities or exposing them to avoidable risk. The differences between HIV and AIDS are also very real in terms of lifestyle implications (such as hospitalisation, medication and social care) and the uncertain timescales between HIV infection and the development of AIDS creates an additional dilemma. The simplified links between sex and AIDS (and illness and death) might be conceptually appropriate for some people with learning disabilities but is also potentially misleading if people do not understand uncertainty or do not have an appreciation of long timescales.

A very challenging example is HIV testing. I would argue that it is not possible to give informed consent for HIV antibody testing (for anyone, with or without a learning disability) without a basic understanding of HIV infection and the differences between being HIV negative or positive (which is what the test indicates) and having an AIDS related illness. Ten key questions help illustrate the argument (with some more complex secondary questions in brackets). These can be used to help to assess informed consent for an HIV test with a person with learning disabilities (Box 3), and relate in part to some of the legal considerations for services identified by Michael Gunn in Chapter 10. There are compelling arguments that such assessments should also give weight to the potential drawbacks of taking an HIV test (Tatchell, 1994). These have been adapted to help further explore questions of informed consent for a person with a learning disability (Box 4).

Box 3
QUESTIONS TO HELP ASSESS INFORMED CONSENT FOR AN HIV TEST

what is a blood test/HIV test? (how it is taken and how long you will have to wait for the result?)

do you know what it shows/tells and does not show/tell you? (do you know it will not tell you if and when you might get AIDS, get ill or die or whether or not you will get HIV or AIDS in the future?)

do you want an HIV test? (why/what reasons?)

do you think you have HIV? (how could you have got it and why?)

how do people get HIV? (and what can people do so they don't get HIV or give it to others?)

how will you feel if you are HIV positive? (what will you do/feel like doing if you are HIV positive/negative?)

how will you feel about having sex and safer sex, relationships and friendships? (now and in the future and telling people)

what happens to someone with HIV? (do you know what AIDS is, how long it may take to get AIDS and what happens to people who have AIDS?)

who would you tell and why? (what do you think they would say/do/think/tell?)

what help and support do you think you will/would need? (in thinking/worrying/coping with HIV/AIDS?)

BOX 4
PROS AND CONS OF HIV TESTING

The Advantages

Knowing your HIV status can help people who have become ill through worry

If you have HIV and get ill, more effective and immediate treatment could result

If you know you are HIV positive you can avoid exposure to other health risks

Having the test can help concentrate priorities and lead to safer sexual choices

You can benefit from regular medical monitoring if you know you are HIV positive

Knowing your HIV status can be empowering for making informed choices

Focusing the mind in relation to safer sex in relationships

The Disadvantages

A positive test does not tell you when you will develop AIDS

A negative test does not guarantee your status (it takes up to six months for antibodies to show up after infection) or protect you from HIV in the future

There are no lasting treatments or cures for HIV or AIDS

Personal trauma and depression may result from a positive test

Problems gaining access to financial services if you are HIV positive (unlikely consequence for a person with a learning disability as they are already largely excluded)

Potential problems with employment and housing (staff support for a person with a learning disability is similarly a potential problem)

Prejudice, abuse and rejection from family and friends may ensue

(adapted from Tatchell, 1994)

17

Responding to Need

Some of the considerations referenced above were used to help inform the content of a set of booklets on HIV and AIDS for people with learning disabilities and their staff and carers (Cambridge, 1996c). The original set made no reference to same sex relationships or sex outside established relationships, with a heterosexual monogamous relationship portrayed as ideal. A balance was struck by also representing homosexuality and casual sex, better matching the messages about HIV and safer sex to the diverse sexual experiences of people with learning disabilities. The possibility of an HIV test was presented as sometimes being a bad idea because of the importance that people are fully aware of its limitations and possible negative consequences for them

The differences between HIV and AIDS were also explained. The booklet on HIV and AIDS produced through self advocacy and peer education in learning disability (People First, 1994) makes similar connections as does an educational package comprising booklets and a video produced by people with learning disabilities (Lawnmowers, 1994). People with learning disabilities constantly receive direct and indirect messages and information about both HIV and AIDS and this ideally needs to be matched to safer sex inputs related to their sexual behaviours and understanding of risk. Simply linking unsafe sex with AIDS and death is neither helpful nor relevant to the sexual lives of many people with learning disabilities.

More careful attention also needs to be paid to the potential risks of HIV infection through oral sex in sex education and training resources in learning disability. Men with learning disabilities are as likely to be in a receptive position in relation to oral sex with men as they are known to be with anal sex (David Thompson explores the reasons for the latter in his chapter). If there is a low risk of HIV from oral sex then it lies in possible transmission through semen and pre cum. Until evidence about the risk of oral transmission to the person sucking is clearer, particularly in relation to other infections like gum disease, then educational resources should have the capacity to address this question and give men and women the information they need to better protect themselves or take more informed risks. The Australian video (FPANSW, 1993) always portrays oral sex with a condom, taking an opposite stance to most British resources, which have tended to prioritise high risk activities such as penetrative anal or vaginal sex in relation to condom use. Neither approach adequately addresses questions of informed choice or risk taking however, although this is difficult to articulate in sex education for people with learning disabilities who may not even have informed choices about sex in the first place.

A decision was also made to use direct words like *fuck*, *suck*, *spunk* and *cock* in the user booklet, because most people know what they mean, even if not culturally appropriate to everyone. Men with learning disabilities in a sex education group were familiar with these words and used them to describe sexual behaviours and body parts. More medical terms like intercourse, semen, oral sex and anus are usually associated with practitioners in positions of authority over people with learning disabilities. Words like fuck are certainly words more able and sexually active people with learning disabilities are likely to know or encounter and should be helped to learn because they are less ambiguous than phrases like doing it or getting on top. People need to be empowered through language to communicate more precisely about consent, body parts, and their preferences for particular sexual behaviours, including safer sex.

Meeting Need

When working on a Department of Health funded HIV risk management resource for men with learning disabilities who have sex with men (Cambridge, forthcoming), ten guiding principles were developed to inform the content and style of the sex educational materials.

1. Present sexuality as positive except in abusive or exploitative situations

2. Show safer sex as empowering

3. Represent the reality of sexual experience of men who have sex with men, including men with learning disabilities

4. Provide explicit images of sex and safer sex and unambiguous language to describe them

5. Include diversity in ethnicity and disability

6. Differentiate between HIV and AIDS in straightforward ways

7. Represent visible aspects of learning disability

8. Minimise irrelevant details and focus on event and place

9. Depict contemporary appearances but also diversity in style

10. Include event sequences, consequences and outcomes

19

The resource has the additional task of addressing a range of possible situations, including cottaging, casual sex and sex with both men and women. In addition to portraying mutual and enjoyable safer sex, it also needed to include abusive and exploitative sex, prostitution and stylised sexual behaviours (Thompson B, 1994) all of which have the potential to impact on men with learning disabilities. Most men with learning disabilities who have sex with men are not in the more fortunate position of gay identified men who can more easily tap into self help groups, informal support networks or dedicated HIV or AIDS services, although gay men often bring their experience to such groups in learning disability.

It was also important to consider what issues such a dedicated resource should address and what it might contain. Practitioners in both HIV and learning disability were consulted and also men in a group sex education setting in learning disability services. The responses confirmed my own interpretations of needs and ways to meet them and are reflected in the staff training materials and specifications for the sex education materials. These include: empowerment to practice safer sex through pictures, words and symbols; acknowledging the differences between HIV and AIDS, timescales and uncertainties; where to get condoms and how to use them effectively; fostering self-image and worth for same sex; showing assertiveness for consenting to sex and saying no to unsafe sex; acknowledging risks and opportunities; representing emotions and feelings; and showing the different places where sex happens.

Micro-organisation and Care Management

It is easy to say that commissioners should undertake needs assessment in HIV and learning disability, design an appropriate array of services to meet identified needs, commission services through contract specification and review effectiveness through monitoring quality and outcomes. It is difficult to articulate this process in relation to specialist learning disability services (HMSO, 1993), let alone sexual health in learning disability. Most people with learning disabilities do not have their sexual, emotional or sexual health needs adequately assessed and identified. Reasons include their lack of meaningful involvement in case reviews and individual planning meetings and lack of power in asserting or communicating their needs and wants. Put this alongside asexual models of service design and delivery and there is a real gap to addressing sexuality and identifying and meeting sexual needs, including safer sex education and other HIV related needs. Commissioners, who are usually responsible for the core tasks of care management, including assessment and individual service planning, must therefore take responsibility for ensuring that sexuality and sexual health are properly represented. Box 5 identifies ten key areas for integrating work on sexuality and HIV into individual programme planning and skill teaching programmes.

BOX 5
KEY AREAS TO BE CONSIDERED IN INDIVIDUAL SERVICE PLANNING

negotiating skills *(negotiating use of condoms and consent to sex and risk)*

expressive and receptive communication skills *(understanding requests and saying or signing yes and no to sex, safer sex and condom use)*

assertiveness skills *(confidence when to say yes and reject unwanted or unsafe situations)*

life skills *(access to condoms and sexual opportunities, including knowledge about HIV and safer sex)*

social skills *(ability to utilise sexual and social opportunities to affect constructive experiences and learning opportunities)*

adaptive behaviour skills *(ability to use condoms properly and effectively during sexual encounters)*

personal presentation skills *(self care and ability to affect positive personal image)*

self-motivation skills *(motivation to protect sexual and emotional health through a positive self-image and self-worth)*

independence skills *(determining own wants and life goals and functional capacity to achieve them)*

personal relationship skills *(capacity and robustness to make and break personal relationships and express emotions)*

Macro-organisation and Joint Working
There needs to be a wider choice of services and resources for meeting different needs, and for service substitution as needs change. It has already been illustrated that expertise is currently localised and that access is restricted. To

achieve this change, commissioners need to adopt a longer term perspective than the usual planning and commissioning cycle. This requires an investment in service development and pump-priming resources to get new specialist services off the ground, and staff training to increase mainstream competence in HIV and sexuality in services for people with learning disabilities. Policy development will similarly be needed and this will have to involve providers and users themselves if policy guidelines are to be effective for managers and practitioners (see Cambridge & McCarthy 1996, for a development model).

Other more familiar disincentives to effective joint commissioning remain. In addition to adopting a short term perspective, agencies tend to minimise the cost or impact to their own budgets. With budgets declining in real terms as well as in relation to specific areas of need, the decision not to provide sex education and safer sex education and counselling in HIV for people with learning disabilities may be easier to make when another agency such as the NHS will have to pick up the tab for the health care consequences of doing nothing. Joint commissioning is potentially no different. Territorial disincentives also remain for many health authorities and social services departments whose boundaries are not coterminous. This makes the development of strategy and integrated services difficult or expensive.

Services and Priorities

Even within a multi-agency approach to sexual health in learning disability there remain barriers between mainstream sexual health services (GUM and HIV testing and counselling), GP purchased services and specialist services working in HIV and learning disability. A solution is to top slice both the learning disability and HIV budgets to protect adequate resources for sexual health in learning disability. With or without ring-fenced budgets, commissioners should consider the following interventions and service models in HIV and learning disability. Preferred options and combinations will depend on local needs and how they are planned to be met.

- specialist sex education through one-to-one work and group workshops (see the work described by David Thompson and Michelle McCarthy in Chapters 5 and 6)
- self advocacy and peer education have proved an effective model in HIV and safer sex education for young people and there are examples of peer education in HIV and learning disability (see work described by Fiona Barber and Paul Redfern in Chapter 8)

- joint projects involving young gay men and men with learning disabilities who have sex with men could also be developed, including befriending and support schemes

- specialist counselling and therapeutic services for people with learning disabilities who are at risk of HIV (see the approach described by Steve Morris in Chapter 7), to cope with issues such as HIV antibody testing, valid consent and confidentiality

- sex education for young people with learning disabilities and parallel training for parents and staff in special schools (see the model explored by David Stewart in Chapter 9)

- training for staff and managers in learning disability services on sexuality and HIV to develop the competence of services, not only to support the sexuality of services users, but on risk assessment and risk management

- specialist training for certain staff to develop key roles and functions within services in relation to sexuality and HIV, such as sex and safer sex education, leading risk assessment and reporting and managing sexual abuse

- policy development on sexuality, including HIV (and sexual abuse), to go hand in hand with staff training and an assessment of user needs. This is necessary to pick up on key practice issues and to develop tailored local responses

- assertiveness training for users, including communication and negotiation skills. This would need to be part of wider work helping people to develop positive self images and to say no to abusive or unsafe sex

- training in learning disability for staff and managers in genito-urinary medicine (GUM), HIV counselling, nursing and other HIV/AIDS provided by the NHS and voluntary organisations

- staff training and sex educational resources which place a priority on risk and convey unambiguous messages about sex and safer sex in relation to the sexual realities and experiences of people with learning disabilities

I would give preference to a dedicated sex education and counselling service, open to referrals from all individuals, agencies and sectors locally and provided free and according to need (HIV and emotional risk). Such a resource would benefit from links with other services such as counselling for sexual abuse and GUM services. I would identify the priority for pro-active providers to develop inhouse competence in management and practice through training and to build safeguards through user involvement such as advocacy and workshops for sex and safer sex education. Both commissioners and providers should share the front loaded costs of consultancy and the direct management and staff time needed to develop the policies and guidelines required to support management and practice. This could well include the costs of developing or accessing specialist services such as those detailed above.

Services and service users would above all benefit from more strategic local approaches, with good multi-agency working, a facilitative and specialist function for health promotion and the integration of social care, health care and educational inputs. This framework should be grounded in a philosophy of empowerment and a culture of delegated responsibility in order to generate innovative, radical and effective service interventions. These should be sensitive to considerations of race, gender, culture and sexuality which are all important for providing appropriate support and responses in HIV and learning disability.

References

Berkelman, R., Thomas P., Kerndt, P., Rutherford G. & Stehr-Green, J. (1989)   *Are AIDS cases among homosexual males levelling? Paper presented at the 5th International Conference on AIDS,* Montreal

Brown, H. & Cambridge, P. (1995)   Contracting for Change: Making Contracts work for People with Learning Disabilities, in (Eds.) T. Philpot and L. Ward, *Values and Visions: Changing Ideas in Services for People with Learning Difficulties,* Butterworth Heineman, London.

Brown, H., Stein, J. & Turk, V. (1995)   *The Sexual Abuse of Adults with Learning Disabilities: Report of a Second Two Year Incidence Survey,* Mental Handicap Research, Vol.8, No.1.

Cambridge, P., Davies, S., Nichol, J., Thompson, D., Morris, S., & Corbett, A . (1994a)
Men with Learning Disabilities who have sex with Men in Public Places, Tizard Centre, University of Kent, Canterbury.

Cambridge, P. (1994)
A Practice and Policy Agenda for HIV and Learning Difficulties, British Journal of Learning Disabilities, Vol.22

Cambridge, P. (1996a)
Men with learning disabilities who have sex with men in public places: mapping the needs of services and users in south east London. Journal of Intellectual Disability Research. Vol.40, No.3.

Cambridge, P. (1996b)
Evaluating Sexual Health Outreach for Women with Learning Disabilities, Bulletin No.15, National Association for the Protection from Sexual Abuse of Adults and Children with Learning Disabilities, University of Nottingham.

Cambridge, P. (1996c)
What You Need to Know about HIV and AIDS, BILD, Kidderminster.

Cambridge, P. (forthcoming)
HIV, Sex and Personal Relationships: a Staff Training and Sex Education Resource with a focus on Men with Learning Disabilities who have Sex with Men, Pavilion, Brighton.

Cambridge, P. & McCarthy, M. (1996)
Developing and Implementing Sexuality Policy for a Learning Disability Provider Service, Health and Social Care in the Community.

Craft, A. (1991)
Living Your Life: a sex education and personal development programme for students with severe learning difficulties, Learning Development Aids, Wisbech.

Davies, P., Hickson, F., Weatherburn, P. & Hunt, A. (1993)
Sex, Gay Men and AIDS, Falmer Press, London.

DoH (1993)

Monitoring and Development: A Special Study of Purchasing and Contracting, Department of Health, London.

Deverell, K. & Rooney, M. (1994)

Using Sexually Explicit Materials for Safer Sex Work with Gay Men, HIV Project, North Thames Regional Health Authority, London.

Dixon, H. (1991)

AIDS and People with Learning Difficulties, BIMH, Kidderminster.

FPANSW (1993)

Feeling Sexy, Feeling Safe, Family Planning Association of New South Wales.

Jones, J. (1993)

Men with Learning Difficulties and Cottaging, Saturday Seminars, North West Thames Regional Health Authority, London.

HMSO (1992)

Community Care: Managing the Cascade of Change, HMSO, London.

HMSO (1993)

Services for People with Learning Disabilities and Challenging Behaviour or Mental Health Needs, HMSO, London.

Kastner, T., Hickman, M. & Bellehumeur, D. (1989)

The provision of services to persons with mental retardation and subsequent infection with HIV, American Journal of Public Health, 79,1-4.

Kastner, T., Nathanson, R. & Marchetti, A .(1992)

Epidemiology of HIV Infection in Adults with Developmental Disabilities, in (Eds.) A. Crocker, H. Cohen & T. Kastner, HIV Infection and Developmental Disabilities, Brookes, London.

King, E.(1993)

Safety in Numbers, Cassell, London.

King, E., Rooney, M., Scott, P. (1992)

HIV Prevention for Gay Men: a Survey of Initiatives in the UK, National AIDS Manual/Gay Men Fighting AIDS/HIV Project/Terrence Higgins Trust.

Kinsey, A. (1948)

Sexual Behaviour in the Human Male, Saunders, Philadelphia.

Lawnmowers (1994)   *The Big Sex Show*, Them Wifies, Newcastle.

LSS (1994)   *Take Care of Yourself: Safer Sex and People with Learning Disabilities*, Lewisham Social Services, London.

McCarthy, M . (1994)   *Against All Odds: HIV and Safer Sex Education for Women with Learning Disabilities*, in (Eds.) L. Doyal, J. Naidoo & T. Wilton, AIDS: Setting a Feminist Agenda Taylor and Francis, London.

McCarthy, M. & Thompson, D. (1992)   *Sex and the 3 Rs: Rights, Responsibilities and Risks,* Pavilion Publishing, Brighton.

McCarthy, M. & Thompson, D. (1994)   *HIV/AIDS and Safer Sex work with People with Learning Disabilities*, in (Ed.) A. Craft, Practice Issues in Sexuality and Learning Disabilities, Routledge, London.

Marneth, A. (1994)   *Geen Kind Meer: Seksuele voorlichting aan jongeren met een verstandelijke handicap vanaf 12 jaar*, Rutgers Stichting, Utrecht.

Morris, S. (1993)   *Protect and Survive,* Community Care, 30 December, 12-13.

Murray, J., MacDonald, R. & Minnes, P. (1995)   *Staff attitudes towards individuals with learning disabilities and AIDS: the role of attitudes towards client sexuality and the issue of mandatory testing for HIV infection*, Mental Handicap Research, Vol.8, No.4, pp321-332

People First (1994)   *Everything you ever wanted to know about Safer Sex but nobody bothered to tell you,* People First, London.

Pink Paper (1992)   *AIDS Budget Slashed*, 214,1 March.

Rooney, M . (1994)   *Information File*, HIV Project, North Thames Regional Health Authority, London.

Simonds, R. & Rogers, M. (1992)   *Epidemiology of HIV Infection in Children and other Populations*, in (Eds.) A. Crocker, H. Cohen & T. Kastner, IIIV Infection and Developmental Disabilities, Brookes, London.

SELHPS (1992) *My Choice, My Own Choice* (video), Pavilion Publishing, Brighton.

Tatchell, P. (1994) *Safer Sexy*, Freedom Editions, London.

Taylor-Laybourn, A. & Aggleton, P. (1992) *HIV Health Promotion Assessment for Men who have Sex with Men in Camberwell*: Final Report, King's Healthcare, London.

THT (1994) *Gay Men' Guide to Safer Sex* (video), Terrence Higgins Trust, London.

Thompson, B. (1994) *Sadomasochism*, Cassell, London.

Thompson, D. (1994) *Sexual Experience and Sexual Identity for Men with Learning Disabilities who have Sex with Men*, Changes, Vol.12, No.4.

Turk, V. & Brown, H. (1993) *The Sexual Abuse of Adults with Learning Disabilities: Results of a Two Year Incidence Survey*, Mental Handicap Research, Vol.6, No.3.

Watney, E. (1993) *Powers of Observation: AIDS and the writing of history, in Practices of freedom*, Rivers Oram, London.

WLHPA (1994) *Piece by Piece* (video), West London Health Promotion Agency, London.

Paul Cambridge is Lecturer in Learning Disability and Service Development Consultant at the Tizard Centre, University of Kent at Canterbury. He has undertaken research on HIV and learning disability and has worked on staff training and policy development in sexuality and learning disability. He is currently developing a staff training and sex education resource with a focus on men with learning disabilities who have sex with men. Prior to 1992, Paul worked in the Personal Social Services Research Unit and in local government.

Chapter 2

The Facts About HIV, Transmission and Treatment

by Jan Welch

History of AIDS

Acquired Immune Deficiency Syndrome (AIDS) was first identified in 1981 in the United States. Cases of Pneumocystis carinii pneumonia, a severe disease which only occurs in immunocompromised people, were identified in groups of people with no apparent reasons for their immune systems to be functioning poorly. AIDS was first decribed in the population of homosexual men and later in haemophiliacs, intravenous drug users and Haitians. Subsequently it was reported from other countries, notably from sub-Saharan Africa where it appeared to be most common in affluent urban heterosexuals.

Initially a variety of causes were suggested, but as more became known about the condition an infection became the leading contender. In 1983 Luc Montagnier's group identified a new retrovirus from a patient with swollen lymph nodes. This virus, now called human immunodeficiency virus type 1 (HIV-1), is generally accepted to be the cause of HIV disease and AIDS.

What is HIV

HIV is one of a group of viruses called retroviruses, which are characterised by the possession of an enzyme called reverse transcriptase. This is a special protein which enables retroviruses to reverse the usual direction of flow of genetic information, by making virus-specific DNA from the RNA of the virus. The new DNA is then inserted into the chromosome of the infected cell in the form of a provirus. This can then be used as a template for the RNA required for virus production. As the provirus has become part of the infected cell it persists within that cell, and in subsequent cells produced from it, resulting in a lifelong infection.

The vast majority of HIV infections worldwide are caused by HIV-1. A slightly different virus, HIV-2, is found in West Africa and occasionally elsewhere. It appears to be milder in its effects, with a longer incubation period.

29

Global Infection

HIV occurs throughout the world. The World Health Organisation (WHO) estimate that by 1994 more than four million AIDS cases had occurred worldwide, with over two thirds of these being in Africa and only 15% in industrialised countries. In the UK, HIV is fortunately still a rare infection except in homosexual and bisexual men and their partners, people who have injected drugs and their partners, and people who have had sexual contact with someone from a part of the world where HIV is common.

HIV infection is an enormous problem for sub-Saharan Africa, resulting in the deaths of many younger wage-earning adults and the orphaning and often also infection of their children. As the result of these factors the life expectancy in Uganda is now only 37 years, the lowest in the world (US Bureau of the Census, 1994).

HIV infection in Africa tends to cluster in urban areas, with transmission following roads. Infection is commonly acquired from commercial sex workers in the hotels and bars of the main towns, and spread onwards by truck drivers and other travellers. Wawer et al. (1991), working in the Rakai district in Uganda, found that more women than men were infected, especially in the roadside trading centres, where 57% of women aged between 20 and 34 had HIV-1. Rural communities are not exempt however. Numm et al. (1994) studied a rural Ugandan community and found that the people most at risk were young married women, with 17.3% of those aged 13-24 having HIV-1. Those women who gave a history of recent genital ulceration were about three times more likely to have HIV.

WHO predict that by the year 2000, there will be a cumulative total of 30 to 40 million cases of HIV, with over 90% in developing countries. By the millennium the majority of new HIV infections in the world are likely to be in Asia, with the largest number of infected people in any single country being in India. The major reported risk factor in India (Jain et al., 1994) is heterosexual contact with commercial sex workers, although injecting drug use is also common in eastern India. Infected blood transfusions may also be a risk factor as paid professional donors are major contributors to the blood supply, of which up to three-quarters is not screened for HIV.

Thailand is another country experiencing a rapid increase in HIV-1 infection. This was fuelled initially by intravenous drug use and commercial sex, but is now spreading rapidly into the general population. Nelson et al. (1994), working in village populations in northern Thailand, found that the prevalence (percentage of people living with HIV infection) more than doubled in two years, from 1.8% in 1990 to 4.6% in 1992.

Transmission of HIV

HIV has been detected in a variety of body fluids, but only blood, semen, vaginal secretions and breast milk have been implicated in transmission. Transmission occurs by sexual contact, injection of blood or blood products, and 'vertically' from mother to child. Although AIDS was first described in homosexual men, whom in many industrialised countries are still the largest infected group, worldwide by far the most common mode of transmission is vaginal intercourse.

HIV is most readily transmitted sexually through penetrative anal sex, with the receptive partner of an HIV-infected man, whether a man or woman, being at most risk. Penetrative anal intercourse with someone with HIV carries a rather lower risk for the insertive partner. In vaginal intercourse, transmission from man to woman is more efficient than from woman to man. Traumatic intercourse, such as may occur in rape or defloration, may increase the risk. Intercourse during menstruation appears to increase the risk for the male partner.

Sexually transmitted diseases markedly increase the likelihood of transmission of HIV infection. This is particularly so for conditions causing genital ulcers, such as syphilis. Circumcision appears to give some protection to both men and their partners.

The ease with which HIV could be spread by the use of contaminated blood or blood products was shown by the presence of AIDS in haemophiliacs early in the course of the epidemic. Since 1985 all blood transfused in the United Kingdom has been screened for HIV, and blood products used in the treatment of haemophilia heat treated. The risk of acquiring HIV from a blood transfusion in the UK is now extremely small, of the order of 1 in a million. Unfortunately this is not the case everywhere as many developing countries cannot afford to screen all blood donations and in addition have to obtain some blood donations from paid donors, who are known to be more likely to have infections than volunteers.

HIV and other blood borne viruses such as hepatitis B and hepatitis C, are readily transmitted by the use of shared needles and equipment by injecting drug users. In Edinburgh the presence of 'shooting galleries' (places where users could buy drugs and share equipment), led to a huge increase in infection during only a few months in 1983. In much of the United Kingdom education about risk reduction and the early institution of needle exchange schemes succeeded in preventing much spread of HIV amongst drug users. Although it is well recognised that injecting drug use frequently occurs amongst prisoners, needle exchange is not currently available in British prisons. In 1993 an outbreak of HIV and hepatitis B infection occurred in Glenochil Prison in Scotland (Taylor et al., 1995). On investigation 33 of 378 inmates reported injecting drugs and of these 12 were HIV antibody positive, with results indicating that at least some had become infected while in prison.

HIV transmission to health care workers is rare but well recognised. It is usually as the result of a needle stick injury, although a few episodes have been described in which blood contaminated broken or inflamed skin. If someone has a needle stick from a needle contaminated by HIV positive blood the risk of them acquiring HIV is about 1 in 270. The use of the antiretroviral drug zidovudine may reduce this risk, but documented transmissions have occurred despite it having been given within a few hours of contact.

Antibodies and the Window Period

Antibodies are complex molecules produced by the body to prevent damage from the presence of a foreign protein or antigen. Detection of antibodies is often used to determine whether someone has been exposed to a specific infection or vaccine. For many infections, such as measles, the presence of antibodies to the measles virus in a well person means that that individual is no longer infected with measles and is immune (will not catch measles again).

HIV is different. The ability of HIV to persist within cells of the immune system means that the presence of antibodies to HIV indicates persisting infection rather than immunity.

Antibodies take time to be produced following infection. In the case of HIV the appearance of antibodies (or 'seroconversion') often takes two or three months and occasionally longer. During this time there may be large quantities of HIV in the blood, with the individual concerned being potentially highly infectious. The gap between infection and seroconversion is known as the window period.

Awareness of the window period is very important in preventing HIV infection. During this time people can readily pass on HIV, before being able to know that they are infected. Safer sexual practices and avoidance of other potential routes of transmission, such as blood donation, are therefore crucial during the period after an episode of risky behaviour.

Sometimes a part of the central core of HIV (the p24 antigen) can be detected before antibodies. Tests to detect p24 antigen are not done routinely but may be useful in making a diagnosis of a seroconversion illness, when characteristically antigen is present but antibodies are not yet detectable.

Infectivity and Disease

Some people with HIV are more infectious, in as much as they are more likely to pass on the infection, than others. Infectivity is related to the amount of virus present in the body fluids. This is termed viral load and is in turn related to the stage of infection. Infectivity is greatest during two periods. First, early in the course of infection, when the virus is present but before antibodies have developed. Second, during late disease, when HIV has overwhelmed the body's defences and is present in large quantities.

HIV damages the body in a number of ways. It causes progressive damage to the immune system, thereby preventing the body from mounting the usual defences against infections and certain tumours. It does this by infecting certain cells which carry on their surfaces a protein called CD4, which HIV uses to gain entry to the cell. The major group of cells which carry CD4 are the CD4 or 'helper' lymphocytes, which are a type of cell found in the white cell part of the blood and in lymph nodes.

The CD4 lymphocytes are important components of the immune system as they orchestrate the way in which the immune system works. HIV infection results in the death of these cells, causing not only increased susceptibility to certain infections as the result of the deficit in 'cell mediated immunity', but also other immunological problems such as allergies.

HIV can also infect other cells which carry the CD4 protein. These include some other cells of the immune system called monocytes and macrophages, which are present throughout the body. Infection of these cells may be responsible for spreading the virus to other parts of the body such as the brain.

33

As well as causing disease as the result of immunosuppression, HIV can also directly damage tissues such as the brain and gut. Both mechanisms commonly contribute to disease.

HIV and AIDS are not synonymous terms. A diagnosis of AIDS is made when an individual has one of a number of infections or tumours which are known to be associated with severe immunodeficiency. The infections are known as 'opportunistic', in that they only occur, or occur in an unusual site or form, when given the opportunity by an inadequate immune system. Many of them are infections which are common but usually cause little or no disease, in people with normal immune systems.

HIV Testing
There are two aspects to testing for HIV: discussion or counselling about the advantages and disadvantages of having the test, and obtaining the correct laboratory result. Discussion about the complex issues involved is commonly carried out by a health adviser or counsellor who has received special training in this area. In the UK, HIV counselling and testing is freely available in departments of genitourinary medicine (sometimes known as GUM clinics or departments of sexual health) of which there is one either within or near every large hospital.

Informed Consent
Having a positive HIV test has profound emotional, social, and financial implications for people, and should not, therefore, be undertaken lightly. Except in very exceptional circumstances, the test should only be carried out with the informed consent of the individual concerned. In law, simply because someone is deemed to be mentally incompetent does not mean that they cannot give consent. The person does, however, need to be fully aware of the consequences of having the test, and this may be very difficult to achieve in someone with a learning disability.

If someone with a learning disability is not able to give informed consent, no-one else can give consent on their behalf. The test could only be carried out if it were deemed to be in the best interests of that individual, and in these circumstances a second, and senior, opinion would be invaluable. If necessary the courts could be approached to give a ruling.

The Blood Test

The blood test for HIV looks for antibodies to HIV, and can usually differentiate between HIV-1 and HIV-2 infection. Before a positive result is released, to ensure that the result is correct, it is usual to confirm it by one or more slightly different tests. Following this, it is good practice to request a second blood sample and test, to ensure that there has not been a labelling error giving an incorrect result.

Although some testing centres offer same day results, it is more usual for the HIV result to take between one day and one week. As positive results need to be given in person, everyone tested is asked to come in to collect their results.

Post-test Counselling

Post-test counselling is essential immediately following a positive HIV result. This should be given by a trained and experienced counsellor; ideally the same person who carried out the pre-test discussion. Post-test counselling usually covers a wide range of issues, including feelings, support, transmission and general precautions, and can be spread over several sessions. Arrangements should also be made for the positive individual to see an HIV physician for assessment and medical advice.

The Natural History of HIV Disease

Most people have no symptoms for years after catching HIV infection. Some people however, experience a so-called 'seroconversion' illness, also known as 'acute primary HIV infection'. This generally occurs a few weeks after acquiring HIV, and is often similar to glandular fever. Common symptoms are fever, fatigue, diarrhoea, swollen lymph nodes and a widespread rash. The illness usually lasts for a couple of weeks, and most people subsequently recover and remain well for some years.

On average it takes 8 - 10 years from acquiring HIV to developing AIDS, but this is quite variable. More rapid transmission is common in people who have received a large quantity of virus, such as in a blood transfusion, in babies who have acquired the infection at or around the time of birth and in older people. Conversely, a small number of others seem to progress very slowly or perhaps not at all. There are still individuals who, by testing stored blood samples, have been shown to have had HIV for fifteen or more years but are still well.

Useful information about an HIV-infected individual's condition can be obtained by taking a blood test to measure the CD4 cell count regularly every three months or so. The CD4 count in people with normal immune systems is usually between about 800 and 1500 and is variable, changing over the course of a day and in response to stresses such as infections. In people with HIV infection the CD4 count tends to decline progressively over the years. As counts can vary considerably, clinical decisions are usually only taken on the basis of more than one count.

While the CD4 count is above 500, HIV-related problems are very unusual and unlikely to develop in the short term. As the count falls much below this, symptoms of disease can start to develop. Early symptoms often relate to the mouth and skin, although some people have other problems such as fatigue, night sweats, or pains in the joints.

Once the CD4 count falls below 200, more serious diseases such as AIDS defining illnesses becomes common. Some conditions, such as Pneumocystis carinii pneumonia (PCP), are common initial presentations of HIV disease, as they can occur at higher counts within this range. Others, such as cytomegalovirus retinitis, an infection which can cause blindness, tend to present much later on, when the CD4 count is below 50.

Persistent generalised lymphadenopathy (PGL) is a common presentation of HIV infection, in which swollen lymph nodes (glands) are present in the neck, armpits and groins. The nodes are characteristically not painful, therefore pain and increasing size should raise concern about other conditions, such as infection or tumour. PGL can present at any stage of HIV infection and does not appear to affect the prognosis of the disease in as much as people with PGL do not develop AIDS faster than others.

Care for People with HIV

In the UK the majority of medical and social care for people who have acquired HIV sexually, is delivered by departments of genitourinary medicine. Such units are generally multi-disciplinary in their approach, with a team comprising doctors, nurses, health advisers and reception staff liaising with social workers, community clinical nurse specialists and general practitioners. The aim is to provide a comprehensive and non-judgemental service which provides optimal support for people living with HIV.

The initial medical assessment includes discussions about the patient's health, a full physical examination, and blood tests to give information about co-existing infections and the functioning of the immune system. A full sexual health check is also offered, in order to identify any other problems.

After the initial visits to the clinic, the frequency of appointments depends on the patient's health. Well people do not generally need to be seen more often than every three months. Once people are symptomatic, the aim is to manage them as out-patients as much as possible, with occasional hospital admissions if necessary. In advanced disease, care is often largely community based, with community clinical nurse specialists, GPs and primary care teams having an increasing role. Hospice admissions can be invaluable for convalescence, respite, and palliative care. Many generic hospices will now accept people with AIDS and in addition there are now a number of specialist hospices for people with HIV disease.

Medical Problems and their Treatment

There are two main aspects to medical treatment for HIV disease. First, the prevention and treatment of opportunistic diseases and second, antiviral treatment.

Other aspects of health care are also important. For example, in late disease severe weight loss is common, but can often be prevented by good dietary advice and support earlier in the course of the disease.

Some opportunistic infections can now be prevented by giving primary prophylactic (preventative) treatment. Primary prophylaxis means that it is given before the individual has experienced the infection. Pneumocystis carinii pneumonia (PCP) is a serious disease which can occasionally be fatal. It can be readily prevented by the use of prophylactic co-trimoxazole (Septrin), given in a low dose. The co-trimoxazole also has an effect in preventing toxoplasmosis of the brain.

When opportunistic infections occur, they need to be treated vigorously, and this often entails an admission to hospital. Subsequently lifelong antibiotic prophylaxis is often required to prevent recurrences of the infection. This is termed secondary prophylaxis, as it is given after an episode of infection has occurred. Box 1 describes the main opportunistic infections associated with HIV disease and AIDS and their treatment.

37

Box I
COMMON OPPORTUNISTIC INFECTIONS

Candidal infection (thrush) can affect the mouth, oesophagus (gullet) or genitals. In the mouth it can cause soreness and sometimes cracks at the angles of the mouth. Inside the mouth white or red patches are usually visible. Oesophageal infection causes pain or discomfort on swallowing. Treatment is straightforward, and consists of antifungal liquid, lozenges to suck or capsules to swallow.

Pneumocystis carinii pneumonia (PCP) used to be a common presentation of HIV disease, but has become much less common since primary prophylaxis with co-trimoxazole has been widely used. PCP causes symptoms of fever, shortness of breath particularly on exertion and dry cough. The symptoms progress over days, weeks or sometimes months. Treatment generally requires admission to hospital for intravenous drugs. Early treatment is important in preventing a fatal outcome or long-term chest problems.

Toxoplasmosis is caused by a small organism, Toxoplasma gondii. The organism is present in raw and undercooked meat, and can also be excreted in the faeces of young cats. In the UK only about one third of people have antibodies to toxoplasmosis, indicating previous exposure, whereas in other countries such as France, most people have been infected. People with HIV who have not been infected with toxoplasmosis can be advised to avoid the infection by eating only well cooked meat and washing their hands thoroughly after contact with cat litter or contaminated earth. When people with toxoplasma and HIV infections become immuno-suppressed the toxoplasma infection can reactivate (become active again) and cause abscesses in the brain. Antibiotic treatment in hospital is usually effective.

Cytomegalovirus retinitis is an infection of the retina (back of the eye) which causes visual disturbances. Without treatment it can lead to blindness. Treatment with antiviral drugs usually needs to be given intravenously, on most days, lifelong. This involves the insertion under anaesthetic of a plastic tube (Hickman line or Portacath) into a large blood vessel. A bag containing the drug to be given can then be connected to the tube each day.

Kaposi's sarcoma (KS) is a tumour which can affect both the skin and internal organs. Firm, pink or purple lumps can be seen on the skin or inside the mouth. They are unsightly and therefore particularly distressing for those affected. KS affecting organs such as the lungs causes progressive symptoms and can be fatal. It is more common in people with HIV who have acquired their infection sexually and is now thought to be related to infection with a newly described herpes virus.

cont.

Unlike a cancer, which generally starts in one site but can spread, KS can start in many different sites at the same time. Removing an individual patch of KS does not therefore, influence the progression of the disease. Treatment for KS is not always necessary, but is given for progressive disease. Radiotherapy is useful for localised areas, and chemotherapy for more generalised disease. Advice on camouflage make-up can be useful if the face is affected.

Lymphoma is a type of cancer of the immune system. In the presence of HIV disease and poor immune function it can be extremely aggressive, although powerful chemotherapy can often produce significant remissions. Common sites affected are the brain, lymph nodes, or intestines.

Antiviral treatment is progressing. At the time of writing (1995) three antiviral drugs are licensed for the treatment of advanced HIV disease. The most widely known of these is zidovudine (AZT). None of the drugs is a cure for the disease, but they may improve symptoms and delay progression. Unfortunately, after any one drug has been taken for a few months, the HIV tends to develop resistance to that drug, with a loss of treatment effectiveness. There is consequently much interest in the use of combinations of antiviral drugs, given together or one after another. It is important that as much information as possible is obtained from the use of combination therapy, particularly when it involves the use of new and promising drugs such as lamivudine (3TC). Studies are therefore designed and run to enable patients to have access to new drug combinations and to find out how effective and well tolerated these are. In the UK entry to such studies can be arranged by most departments of genitourinary medicine.

Women and HIV

Women with HIV have special problems, both medical and social. Women are often emotionally, financially and socially dependent on men, both for themselves and for their children. Dependence makes negotiation difficult or impossible and so may be a major barrier to safer sexual practices, such as condom use.

The progression of HIV infection is generally similar in men and women. A major exception is Kaposi's sarcoma, which is rare in women except those coming from sub-Saharan Africa.

A major determinant of prognosis is access to health care. In the UK everyone with HIV should in theory have equal access to medical care with the National Health Service. In practice this is not always so, particularly for women who lack assertiveness skills enabling them to identify the best care for themselves, whose first language is not English, or who have lifestyles which make it difficult for them to keep hospital appointments.

Abnormal cervical smears are more common in women with HIV than those without. Cervical smears detect cells which indicate an increased risk of cervical cancer developing over the next 10-20 years. As yet studies have not shown an increased risk of symptomatic cervical cancer in women with HIV, but women with HIV are advised to have yearly smears and further assessment (colposcopy) and treatment if any abnormality is found.

Mother to child transmission of HIV is an important consideration as many women with HIV wish to have babies. The presence of HIV infection may not reduce this desire, but instead make the women concerned keener to experience childbearing within their limited lifespan. Improved understanding of how infection is passed from mother to child has made it possible to reduce the risk of this significantly. This makes it especially important to identify women with HIV before or during pregnancy, in order that interventions and support can be offered.

Although transmission of HIV from mother to baby (vertical transmission) can probably occur at any time during pregnancy, most transmission occurs at birth or as the result of breast feeding. Only a minority of women with HIV pass the infection on to their babies. The European Collaborative Study (1992) looked at 721 children born to 701 mothers. Overall 14% of babies were infected. The risk of infection was related to the mother's health; only 6% of women with normal CD4 cell counts passed on the infection to their babies, whereas 31 % of women with AIDS did so. The study confirmed previous reports that breast feeding is a very efficient way of transmitting HIV, more than doubling the risk.

The mode of delivery may also be important. A later publication from the European Collaborative Study (1994) suggested that caesarean section approximately halved the risk. This finding has been questioned by the results of other studies, however.

A highly promising approach to reducing transmission is the use of antiviral drugs such as zidovudine. In the AIDS Clinical Trials Group (ACTG) 076 (Connor et al., 1994) protocol zidovudine was given to women with HIV during pregnancy, and to their babies for six weeks after birth. This showed a reduction in vertical transmission from 25.5% for the babies of women given placebo treatment to only 8.3% for the babies whose mothers (and they themselves) received zidovudine.

The presence of HIV antibody in a baby born to a woman with HIV does not necessarily mean that the baby is infected, as the mother's antibodies can cross the placenta into the baby's bloodstream. If the baby is not infected, the HIV antibodies will gradually disappear, but this may take up to eighteen months. New tests, which look for the presence of genetic information from HIV, can be invaluable in determining whether a baby is infected earlier than this. Establishing earlier that a baby is uninfected is helpful in reducing the mother's anxiety, as well as allowing the baby's primary prophylaxis against PCP to be stopped.

Condoms are extremely helpful in reducing HIV transmission. They are less effective in preventing pregnancy and so the ideal for women with HIV who do not wish to become pregnant is to use another method of contraception as well. No method of contraception is ideal. Combined oral contraceptives suit many women, but need to be taken regularly to be effective. The progesterone only pill has even more exacting requirements, which are difficult for most women with HIV to manage. Long-acting injectable contraceptives are an excellent choice for many women, although sometimes irregular bleeding results, which may increase the risk of HIV transmission as well as being debilitating for the woman concerned. The intra-uterine contraceptive device may increase the risk of pelvic infection, but for some women may be the easiest sustainable option.

41

Appendix

Classification of HIV infection

This is the classification system currently used in the UK (adopted 1993).

Category A

Acute (primary) HIV infection
or
Asymptomatic HIV infection
or
Persistent Generalised Lymphadenopathy

Category B

Symptomatic with conditions other than those in A or C attributed to HIV infection or which indicate a defect in cell mediated immunity eg:
• oral candidiasis (thrush of the mouth)
• candidiasis of the female genitals which is persistent, frequent, or poorly responsive to treatment
• symptoms such as fever or diarrhoea lasting> 1 month
• hairy leukoplakia (white patches in the mouth caused by a persistent viral infection)
• herpes zoster (shingles) if recurrent or extensive

Category C

Clinical conditions categorised as AIDS
eg:
• candidiasis of the oesophagus
• cervical cancer
• cryptococcal meningitis
• cryptosporidiosis, with diarrhoea for> 1 month
• cytomegalovirus retinitis
• encephalopathy (dementia) due to HIV
• herpes causing ulcers for> 1 month
• Kaposi's sarcoma
• lymphoma
• tuberculosis
• pneumocystis carinii pneumonia (PCP)
• toxoplasmosis of the brain
• wasting syndrome (weight loss of >10% over baseline, with no other cause), and 30 days or more of either diarrhoea or weakness with fever

References

Connor, E.M., Sperling,R.S., Gelber, R., Kiseley, P., Scott, G., O'Sullivan, M.J., VanDyke, R., Bey, M., Shearer, W., Jacobson, R., Jimenez, E., O'Neill, E., Bazin, B.,Delfraissy, J-F, Culnane, M., Coombs, R., Elkins, M., Moye, J., Stratton, P., & Balsley, J.(1994) — *Reduction of maternal-infant transmission of human immunodeficiency virus type 1 with zidovudine treatment*, New England Journal of Medicine, 331, pp.1173-80.

European Collaborative Study (1992) — *Risk factors for mother-to-child transmission of HIV-1*, Lancet, 339, pp.1007-12.

European Collaborative Study (1994) — *Caesarean section and risk of vertical transmission of HIV-1 infection*, Lancet, 343, pp.1464-1467.

Jam M.K., John T.J., & Keusch G.T. (1994) — *A review of human immunodeficiency virus in India*. Journal of Acquired Immune Deficiency Syndromes, 7, pp.1185-1194.

Nelson, K.E., Suriyanon, V., Taylor, E., Wongchat, T., Kingkeow, C., Srirak, N., Lertsrimongkol, C., Cheewawat, W. & Celentano, D. (1994) — *The incidence of HIV-1 infections in village populations of northern Thailand*, AIDS, 8, pp.951-955.

Numm A.J., Kengeya-Kayondo, J.F., Malamba, S.S., Seeley, J.A., & Mulder, D.W. (1994) — *Risk factors for HIV-1 infection in adults in a rural Ugandan community: a population study* AIDS, 8, pp.81-86.

Taylor, A., Goldberg, D., Emslie, J., Wrench, J., Gruer, L., Cameron, S., Black, J., Davis, B., McGregor, J., Follett, E., Harvey, J., Basson, J. & McGavigan, J. (1995) — *Outbreak of HIV infection in a Scottish prison* British Medical Journal, 310, pp.289-292

Wawer, M.J., Serwadda, D. & Musgrave, S.D., — *Dynamics of spread of IIIV 1 infection in a rural district of Uganda*, British Medical

Konde-Lule, J.K.,   Journal, 303, pp.1303-1306.
Musagara, M. &
Sewankambo, N.K .(1991)

US Bureau of the   *Center for International Research, Population*
Census (1994)   *trends, Uganda* (Washington, US Bureau of
                                    the Census).

Jan Welch is Consultant Genito-Urinary Physician at King's Healthcare NHS Trust in South East London. She is particularly interested in the care of women with HIV and, in conjunction with paediatricians, runs a family clinic for women and children infected and affected by HIV. She also leads a multi-disciplinary team which includes doctors, nurses, health advisers and associated professionals, which aims to deliver high quality holistic care.

Chapter 3

HIV Prevention and Health Promotion

By James Nichol

This chapter looks at ways in which HIV prevention and sexual health programmes in health promotion services can respond to the needs of people with learning disabilities, their carers and service providers.

Given the often confused and superficial understanding of health promotion as an activity, the specialism is first explained by reviewing the different theoretical positions adopted. Each position represents a different interpretation of the health promotion task and of the kinds of practical interventions most likely to be appropriate and effective. These are identified as they form the basis for assessing different practical approaches. This analysis is then used to inform an account of the work carried out by Health First, the specialist provider agency for health promotion in the inner London boroughs of Lambeth, Lewisham and Southwark.

Attention is therefore paid to the evolving philosophy of the work, as the agency learned more about what was needed, the forms of 'healthy alliance' created with specialist agencies, carers and service users, and the types of project enabled by the relationships and working methods which developed. It is demonstrated that mainstream health promotion services can play an important part in supporting the sexual health and development of people with learning disabilities when both the political will and financial resources are available.

Defining Health Promotion

Health promotion specialists have developed a number of conceptual tools to anchor their understanding of the health promotion function. The field of health promotion can be divided into three basic (but overlapping) activities, namely education, prevention and health protection.

Health education is classically described as 'communication activity aimed at enhancing well-being and preventing or diminishing ill-health in individuals

45

and groups, through favourable influencing of the knowledge, beliefs, attitudes and behaviour of those with power and the community at large' (Tannahill, 1985). The belief of this statement is that education is not only directed at those whose own health is at stake, but also at anyone who might influence the situation, thereby recognising that at least some of the significant blocks to understanding may not lie with the population most at risk. Proponents of this approach suggest that 'upwards' education, from service users to service providers to funding bodies, is essential. The assumption is that given space and support in exploring and articulating their needs, it is the people whose health is at issue who have the best understanding of what those needs are.

Prevention specifically focuses on disease and other unwanted states, such as HIV infection and AIDS. In wider sex education with people with learning disabilities, this may well also focus on contraception and the prevention of unwanted pregnancy. It either has to do with preventing the state entirely or with mitigating its effects. It therefore involves measures like immunisation. Given the absence of the immunisation option in HIV, the first thought is often to concentrate on telling men to wear condoms during penetrative sex as a kind of less reliable substitute for the absent medical technology. The temptation in this context is to define health education narrowly as providing information in support of a prevention programme focused around one identified behaviour change. The prevention task on its own does not necessarily involve looking at the context of people's lives and is therefore an important but incomplete form of health promotion.

Health protection has been defined as 'legal or fiscal controls, other regulations or policies, or the positive enhancement of well-being' (Tannahill, 1985). Health regulation measures can therefore range from procedures concerning the provision of condoms in residential homes, through the creation and review of relationship and sexuality policies for agencies delivering care in the community for people with learning difficulties, to major legal and social measures like age of consent laws and benefit levels. All are likely to exert some influence on health and well-being, including a host of legal and quasilegal measures which might well be health-negative in their effects. The latter also need to be looked at as areas for possible health promotion activity.

Two other key terms need to be examined. The first is 'self-empowerment'. This has been identified (Tones, 1981) as a discreet approach to health education with the aim of facilitating the kind of informed choice which was earlier (when discussing a purely information giving approach to health education) seen as an illusory goal. The main difference in approach is that steps are taken to enhance the self-esteem and autonomy of clients through the techniques of personal development work, such as assertiveness training. Empowerment has been seen to have the similar aim to 'improve health by developing people's ability to understand and control their health status to whatever extent is possible within their environmental circumstances' (French & Adams, 1986). Examples of methods used include life and social skills training and self-empowerment to support the negotiation of safer-sex. Aggleton (1991) reports studies from the USA showing that work involving group discussion and role play has at least generated a more positive attitude towards safer sex, even if behaviour change is more difficult to demonstrate.

The second term is 'community development'. Within the context of health promotion, community can be defined as a network of people linked by where they live, the work they do, their ethnic background and other factors they have in common (Ewles & Simnett,1985). The networks may be formal or informal, therefore the important point to note is that communities are considered to have a collective capacity to respond to health issues. Community development is therefore the process of developing that capacity. It can begin with the expressed needs of the community itself, or it may involve health workers catalysing a sense of community where none existed before. The goal may be to raise levels of awareness about specific health issues or to increase confidence within the community, leading to demands for major changes in resources and systems. The distinctive feature of community development is that it emanates from the specific shared experience of an identified group of people working together. The role of gay men in creating a culture of safer sex promotion and practice in relation to HIV is an outstanding example of such work.

Strategy and Belief

Given the sort of territory which health promotion occupies, strategies for intervention will depend not only on the problems to be addressed but also on the fundamental beliefs both about health and about the status and role of different groups in society (whether service user or service provider). In this context it is usual to talk about models of health promotion, but a more searching approach has been to think about the place which different strategies occupy on a 'paradigm map' (Figure 1).

The paradigm map concept in health promotion (and also in the contexts of counselling, social work and social research) has primarily been developed by Ray Holland of King's College, London (1990). Holland's map uses two dimensions to define spaces (or paradigms) each representing a way of thinking, seeing or feeling about the world. As the paradigms represent fundamentally different assumptions and interpretations, they generate different ideologies and so different professional practice and working methods.

The vertical axis represents the degree to which societies are seen as well-ordered (requiring fine-tuning and regulation) or as dysfunctional (requiring radical transformation). The horizontal axis distinguishes objective and subjective forms of knowledge. Four positions result from using each dimension as an axis on a graph. These four paradigms are described for reference in Boxes 1 to 4.

Box I
THE FUNCTIONALIST PARADIGM

Functionalism is an objective approach based on an acceptance of social norms, a commitment to medical forms of intervention and valuing medical practitioners as professionals whose expert advice we should all heed. The underlying assumption is that individual behaviour is the main cause of ill-health and that individuals have freedom to choose 'health' life-styles. The resulting 'medical' or 'behaviour change' model (Ewles & Simnett, 1985), is one in which health experts decide what populations need to do and provide messages about the changes in individual behaviour necessary to accomplish these goals. Some attention is paid to environmental and legislative/regulatory factors (concern about the spread of HIV legitimised the advertising of condoms on TV). The chief emphasis is on individual responsibility, with the professional role unabashedly directive in information and advice. This is the position of the Department of Health's major policy statement on health promotion *The Health of the Nation* (DOH, 1992). This approach has been institutionally dominant and widely criticised in the professional literature (Ewles & Simnett, 1985) which has questioned the assumption that individual behaviour is the main cause of illhealth and that individuals have genuine freedom to choose 'healthy' life-styles. The assumption is that the expert knows best, despite the fact that experts are known to disagree and change their minds, for example, about barrier protection for oral sex. The imposition of values involved and the danger of inducing guilt in people has also led to this approach being characterised as victim-blaming, hierarchical and elitist (French & Adams, 1986) or as lacking evidence on effectiveness (Tones, 1981).

BOX 2
THE HUMANIST APPROACH

This continues to accept social norms, but validates the subjective experience of individuals, attempting to relate to people within their own worlds. There is greater acceptance that people have different individual needs because they belong to diverse communities and cultures with different life experiences and perspectives. With this awareness, health promotion interventions tend to be more sensitive by paying more attention to the meaning of health in the context of the conflicting priorities of life. Before talking about safer sex, the health promoter would comprehend what concepts like 'safe' and 'sex' really mean to people and how HIV prevention fits with people's existing feelings, experience and knowledge of sex. For this reason, most of those concerned with HIV prevention for people with learning disabilities have been at pains to place their work in the much larger context of exploring personal relationships and sexuality, rather than focusing on narrow health messages that might otherwise seem irrelevant.

The humanist position is also willing to show some scepticism about the role of professionals (Holland, 1990). Professionalism is no longer seen as a neutral and scientific concept but as an interest group within the operations of society. The humanist position, like the functionalist, takes the world as it finds it but precisely through a willingness to engage with subjectivity, it becomes more questioning and relativist and less value-laden.

BOX 3
THE RADICAL HUMANIST PERSPECTIVE

This takes the honouring of subjective experience a stage further, by perceiving the effects of social pressures on individuals and communities more clearly, with existing society seen as a source of depowerment, stunting the development of human potential. Institutions concerned with health and care are themselves seen as problematic, disguising the real nature of their users' difficulties concerning their own health and welfare. Services are seen to deny user groups their own initiative and to oppress them through the creation of a 'learned helplessness' and dependency, falsely construed and presented as support. Ivan Illich famously referred to the helping professions in health, welfare and education as disabling. Service users, especially those from vulnerable and marginalised communities such as people with learning disabilities are seen as being systematically taught to believe in their own dysfunction and incompetence.

Those who support the radical humanist position often argue that the authentic role of professionals is not to empower service users, but to avoid disempowerment and provide space for healing to take place. Work on sexual health would be seen as a project of healing wounds created by the absence of supportive sex education in childhood and compounded by oppressive messages about gender roles and sexual preference. It might also involve working with deeper wounds created by child and adult sexual abuse, a common experience for both women and men with learning disabilities.

Box 4
THE RADICAL STRUCTURALIST APPROACH

This perceives society as oppressive and dysfunctional and attempts to look at this objectively, developing a science of society which gives an account of this condition. Drawing on Marxist and feminist traditions, the radical structuralist sees social oppression as fundamental and as objectively determined in both the economic /material and emotional/sexual spheres. A fully successful culture of health promotion would therefore be directly linked to the ending of those oppressions, for example in terms of disability and sexual orientation, although class and ethnicity would also be factors for many people with learning disabilities. Health promotion initiatives would involve the mobilisation, or better the self mobilisation, of communities to create the maximum amount of beneficial social change, campaigns aimed at legislative and institutional reform and the seeking of alliencies for wider social transformation. The primary focus might be on raising sexual self-esteem and enriching sexual experience in the context of genuinely aware choice on safer sex/sexual health and on challenging the social, institutional and legal blocks in these areas. But the overall goal would concern a much wider emancipation.

The starting point was a local health promotion initiative. In January 1990 the South East Thames Regional Health Authority (SETRHA) organised a conference on HIV and people with learning disabilities (SETRHA, 1990) which concluded that 'given the spread of HIV and the increasing number of people with learning difficulties in the community, attention needs to be focused on the ways in which they are particularly vulnerable'.

Research in the UK and elsewhere (Brown & Craft, 1989), had already demonstrated a high incidence of sexual abuse among people with learning disabilities and there is a known relationship between the history of sexual abuse and a propensity to HIV risk behaviour. People with learning disabilities were presenting with unwanted pregnancies and sexually transmitted diseases and a small number were known to have developed AIDS, some of whom had died. Local discussions following the conference revealed a dearth of sex education, including work on self-esteem and relationship issues, together with a lack of confidence and perceived support among carers and trainers. A need for appropriate educational resources was also identified, given the inaccessibility of mainstream written and audio-visual messages to most people with learning disabilities.

The conference brought together people working in the fields of learning disability and HIV prevention/health promotion and demonstrated a clear need for health promotion intervention of some kind. Questions still remained on the nature of optimal intervention, including issues of strategy, multi-agency collaboration and prevailing beliefs about the nature of the health promotion task.

Learning and Evolving
In 1990 the West Lambeth Health Promotion Department was a small sub-unit of the then West Lambeth Health Authority's Public Health Department. In common with most health promotion departments linked to the old District Health Authorities, its remit included a responsibility for HIV prevention work among local communities. People with learning disabilities were first identified as a possible target group for work on HIV prevention and sexual health in the middle of 1990. The decision was essentially a product of the South East Thames conference and its other regional counterparts. The health promotion task was framed initially in prevention terms, though it was already clear that a purely information giving and behaviour change message would not be adequate to meet the needs of the target population. People in the learning disability community were clear that a simple top down safer sex message would not be meaningful. In order to make any intervention that was credible, a health promotion specialist would need to depart from the understandings of the functionalist paradigm of the institutional public health culture while preserving support and funding for the programmes.

Melissa Fenton (1989) argues that people with disabilities are depowered by society in specific ways and that many are treated as second-class citizens. Negative attitudes are deeply inbred within our culture and adults with learning disabilities are still citizens who should live and function as an integral part of the community. Health Authority funding, negotiated by the Health Promotion Department with its own paymasters, depended on an explicit adoption of HIV prevention as the main aim. However, the project was following aims and using methods desired by many people in the self-advocacy movement for people with learning disabilities. Health promotion, with access to HIV prevention funds, was able to provide resources and person power for the project. The approach was to explore choice of sexual issues, and by the early part of 1991 it had identified three main ways of doing this: two in the sphere of health education and one in the sphere of health protection.

51

Resource Development

The first was a review of education resources and a commitment to promote the use of existing good resources. By 1991 there were already a number of specialist resources available, but still many obvious gaps. In particular, Empower identified the lack of an appropriate and accessible video and training pack that would introduce the main relationship and sexual health issues relevant to HIV prevention. In March 1991 a decision was taken to try to fill this gap with a video and teaching pack which would incorporate a number of features.

The resource would make two main points in 25 minutes: the value of strong validation and support for someone exploring their sexual options and a clear message in a relevant context about the use of condoms for penetrative sex. Together with the teaching pack, it would also provide opportunities for facilitators to bring out other issues including sexual preference, roles, assertiveness, alternatives to penetrative sex and relations with parents and professionals. The video would use a TV soap format as a comfortable and user-friendly medium for large numbers of people with learning disabilities. It would deliberately model the optimistic resolution of problems (as a contradiction to the gloomy messages that sometimes seem to overwhelm the subject). The teaching pack would suggest activity-based sessions that could be related back to defined scenes from the story and which could be used by relatively inexperienced facilitators in group homes, day centres, Gateway Clubs and other settings.

The ideas came quickly and a script was commissioned by Southside Partnership, one of the agencies most involved with Empower, as a marketing tool for substantive funding. This was granted by the, then, South East London Commissioning Agency in April 1992 (District Health Authorities having just been abolished) and the video was launched with the title *My Choice, My Own Choice* (SELHPS, 1992) on World AIDS Day (1 December 1992). In this case, the funds were given to the South East London Health Promotion Service (SELHPS), of which the West Lambeth Health Promotion Department had now become a part. SELHPS organised the tendering process for a video production company and the ongoing relationship with the successful company, *First Field*. It also undertook the commissioning, editing and publication of the teaching pack, using in house facilities for graphics.

Education and Training

The second Empower initiative was the development and testing of educational programmes on personal relationships and sexuality for people with learning disabilities, service managers, staff groups in statutory and voluntary agencies (mainly residential homes and day centres) and parents' groups. Members of Empower were actively treated as though they were children with no need or right to be sexually active with partners 'in general, society does not encourage people with learning disabilities and/or physical disabilities to become more independent'. One effect of this is to make people more vulnerable to sexual abuse and relatively careless of their own safety.

As a consequence, meaningful work on safer sex with people with learning disabilities requires a culture change for the whole community, including carers and the service managers and workers involved with them. The recognition that sexual identity and needs must first be acknowledged and supported by that wider community induces a paradigm shift to at least radical humanism, with the recognition of a need for collective change if people with learning disabilities are to have a realistic chance of practicing safer sex.

The specific role of the specialist health educator within this framework involves extending the confidence, skills and personal development of professionals, carers and service users in dealing with sexual issues as well as providing information on HIV and sexual health. Moving from a philosophical basis of radical humanism, the model of intervention would involve self-empowerment within a framework of community development. In this case, the community is seen to include carers (usually parents) and professionals because the lives and choices of these people and those with learning difficulties are so obviously intertwined. It is however, also clear that a community so defined is one in which different interests exist because the parties do not enjoy equal relationships and are not grounded in the same experiences.

Creating 'Empower'

This thinking led to the creation of 'Empower', the Lambeth Working Group on Relationships and Sexuality for People with Learning Difficulties. This body principally comprised professionals and carers in the field of learning disability in the statutory and voluntary sectors. It also included health promotion specialists and at times, other health workers. It was officially a sub-group of the Lambeth Joint Planning Team for Services for People with Learning Difficulties, a multi-agency body whose overall task was to oversee service provision in the borough and in particular to implement the Community Care Act. In its original form Empower did not include user representation. Initially, the group had three objectives.

1. to ensure the availability of appropriately presented information on HIV and sexual health to people with learning disabilities

2. to provide appropriate training and support to individuals and organisations living and working with people with learning disabilities on relationships and sexual health including HIV

3. to promote the development of work with people with learning disabilities that would enable them to negotiate safer practices on their own terms.

It could be argued that Empower was not a pure community development project because it was not user-directed, even when user is interpreted in the wide sense of engaged in running such programmes in a variety of contexts: adult education, group homes, day centres, clubs and other voluntary settings. At first the health promotion input was to provide resources and teaching aids and sometimes venues.

Later, the West Lambeth and Camberwell Health Promotion Departments (both eventually subsumed into SELHPS and eventually Health First) were involved in running staff training programmes in particular linked to the overall work of Empower (at that time restricted to the London Borough of Lambeth). West Lambeth specifically undertook a number of programmes for Lambeth Social Services and other local agencies, mainly based on an eight half day format. There were also two initiatives for parents, each on a series of eight evenings, one in conjunction with Lambeth Contact-a-Family and the other with Lambeth mencap. One result of the Empower initiative was the enhanced networking that enabled people to meet and work together in a variety of agencies, enabling the overall level of educational activity to be high, echoing the multi-agency 'healthy alliance' approach.

Policy Development

The third activity was an endeavour to generate an appropriate set of policies and guidelines on the right to sexual expression, to be adopted by all the agencies working in Lambeth and to accompany these with effective mechanisms for implementation and the provision for specialist support where necessary.

From the outset, Empower discussions emphasised the need to move away from the production of a purely paper policy. The concern was that an instant policy would on its own do nothing to promote the kind of culture change deemed necessary to achieve the sexual health goals being sought, rather than a living and evolving approach to policy.

The eventual solution recommended by Empower and adopted by the Joint Planning Team was to create the Lambeth Advisory Group on Personal Relationships and Sexuality for People with Learning Difficulties, which did have user representation, to draft an outline policy containing key principles to which all Lambeth agencies would sign up. The Advisory Group would then remain in business to assist individual agencies in producing detailed guidelines to meet their own needs. The advisory group would remain on hand to assist with implementation, provide specialist support and contacts and monitor the success of the policy.

Further Evolution

At the beginning of 1993, Empower underwent a change of direction. The video had been produced, the educational profile in Lambeth had been raised and the Lambeth Advisory Group had been created to deal with policy work. Health Promotion was one of the agencies represented on this group. Empower itself broadened its scope to cover Lambeth, Southwark and Lewisham and had another three tasks. The first was the local promotion of the video, made available by agreement with the funders, for £10 to agencies in the three boroughs. Health promotion became the local vendor of *My Choice, My Own Choice*. It also undertook a series of one day training programmes for facilitators wishing to use the resource.

The second task was to look at ways in which the impact of training could be increased. Service-based staff training was not always sufficient to help services take on the issues with confidence and many providers continued to be reticent. Some people felt that the necessary skill-building and culture change would be too difficult in some agency settings and that specialist organisations promoting personal development work or forms of peer education would be more successful. During this period Empower offered occasional half-day sessions on particular teaching points, taking motivated staff members out of their work setting to explore specific issues.

Members of SELHPS supported a series of workshops on HIV/Hep B and learning difficulty organised by the Tizard Centre at the University of Kent on behalf of the South East Thames Regional Health Authority (Cambridge, 1994). These were aimed at managers of learning disability services in the region as a whole. Overall, health promotion specialists undertook less direct training but continued to finance trainers and facilitators from other agencies.

The third new initiative derived from the discussion, at that time becoming more widespread in the field, about men with learning difficulties who cottage. Anecdotal evidence suggested that numbers of men were placing themselves at risk of HIV infection in these settings. The problem was difficult to assess because of a lack of knowledge and the barriers, both ethical and practical, to obtaining it. To begin, it was decided to seek funds to commission local research into the issue (as a needs assessment exercise). The research would be based on the collection of information from services, using methods which made it impossible to identify individual service users.

Assessing Needs

Funding was secured from the local health commissioner and a steering group for the work was set up. This comprised the Director of Southside Partnership, a health promotion specialist from SELHPS, David Thompson from the AIDS Sex Education Team at Harperbury Hospital (who had existing experience of working with service users who cottage), El Corbet from Respond and Paul Cambridge from the Tizard Centre (who was responsible for research). Other members took on related functions. David Thompson led a training day on the topic.

The survey was published, together with a record of the training day towards the end of 1993 (Cambridge et al., 1993), which discusses the resistance and other difficulties experienced. Anecdotal evidence from the training day for people who work with men with learning disabilities who cottage, confirmed the particularly high HIV risk in this context. This is because sex in cottages involving men with learning disabilities is more frequently penetrative with decisions about condoms left to the discretion of the more able and powerful man. HIV risk and abuse may be carried over to other partners, especially if they are women with learning disabilities who occupy an even lower place on the hierarchy of oppression.

The Final Stages

It was hoped to use the survey evidence to demonstrate the need for funding initiatives to support men with learning disabilities who cottage, education and awareness for service providers and improving specialist services through one-to-one health education, counselling and group work. It was also thought that the work would encourage an increased sense of urgency concerning work on relationships and sexuality with people with learning disabilities.

This failed to materialise and although considerable public funding was now being given to men who have sex with men, men with learning disabilities were seen as a minority within the minority. The local health commissioner had provided substantial funds for making *My Choice, My Own Choice* and may have felt that a sufficient contribution had been made to the learning disability field with this nationally successful resource. This contrasted with the belief of Empower and the health promotion specialists, that the video was in reality a rather gentle introduction to issues of relationships and safer sex for people who had not previously worked through them. Using in part the evidence from the needs assessment work, Paul Cambridge has since secured funding from the Department of Health for an integrated sex education and staff training resource on HIV and learning disability, with a focus on men who have sex with men.

Conclusions

On a pragmatic level, the Empower initiative resulted from the merging of two agendas. One was increasing concern within the learning disability community that relationships and sexuality should be properly addressed. It flowed from the conviction that people with learning disabilities should have the same rights and opportunities as other adults, especially now that there was a commitment to supporting them in the community rather than in closed institutions. The second agenda was the public health campaign for HIV prevention, which was well funded and which sought to extend its reach to target populations deemed to be disadvantaged or at particular risk. An opportunity arose for health promotion because both agendas could be met through a common strategy beyond a focus on simplified safer sex messages.

From an HIV prevention perspective, there was an imperative to move away from the functionalist paradigm of health promotion, even though this was most widely understood within the health service as a whole. Fortunately, both the traditions of health promotion as a specialism and of HIV activism provided an awareness of alternative models. The evolution to a humanistic and implicitly radical perspective was swift and reasonably acceptable. Short term, it was possible to generate and fund a significant work programme but longer term blocks emerged partly as a consequence of reorganisations within the health promotion service.

One choice was a further paradigm shift, taking on board more fully and explicitly the insights of the radical humanist perspective by addressing the agenda of radical structuralism. The alternative was to say that the health promotion service had already done as much as it could. In the event, the position of the health promotion service itself within the NHS culture and funding structure placed constraints on its philosophical evolution. At the same time, a local redirection and re-assessment of HIV prevention funding (focused more on the high risk groups in the epidemic, with message maintenance strategies targeted on easily accessible settings), seemed to make people with learning disabilities, including men who cottage, once more a low priority group. In terms of overall resources, it could be argued that the learning disability community had already had its share of what was available and that the resources were now needed elsewhere. What such an argument ignores is the lost potential for the further evolution of an increasingly knowledgeable, confident and mature project which had reached the point of breakthrough into challenging and important forms of work.

The Empower project emerged from a situation in which a number of interested groups and agendas within them coalesced happily and were able to achieve practical results. When the interest groups and their agendas began to separate, the specialist health promotion service was institutionally too weak to remain a focus for the work. It did however help to prepare the ground for others more favourably situated to take the work forward. One of the tasks of the health promoter is to be a catalyst. In this sense, the Empower project can claim a measure of success.

References

Aggleton, P. (1991)   *HIV/AIDS health promotion - past, present and future.* Royal Society of Medicine AIDS Letter, 25.

Brown, H. &   *Thinking the Unthinkable (papers on sexual abuse and people*
Craft, A. (1989)   *with learning difficulties)* (1989) H. Brown and A. Craft (Eds.). London: FPA Education Unit.

Cambridge, P., *Men with Learning Difficulties who have Sex with Men in*
Davies, S., Nichol, J., *Public Places.* SELHA needs assessment project report.
Thompson, D., Morris Canterbury: CAPSC.
S. & Corbett, A (1993)

Cambridge, P. (1994) *A Practice and Policy Agenda for HIV and Learning Difficulties*, British Journal of Learning Disabilities. Vol 22

DoH (1992) *The Health of the Nation: A Strategy for Health in England,* Presented to Parliament by the Secretary of State for Health. London: HMSO.

Ewles, L. & *Promoting Health: A Practical Guide to Health Education.*
Simnett, I. (1985) Chichester: Wiley.

Fenton, M.. (1989) *Passitivity to Empowerment: A Living Skills Curriculum for People with Learning Disabilities.* London: Radar.

French, J. & *Theories of health education.* Health Education Journal, 45,
Adams, L. (1986) (2), p.71-74.

Holland, R. (1990) *The paradigm plague: Prevention, cure and inoculation.* Human Relations, 43, (1), p.23-48.

SELHPS (1992) *My Choice, My Own Choice*, a First Field production for the South East London Health Promotion Service in conjunction with Southside Partnership London: SELHPS. Distributed by Pavilion Press: Brighton.

SETRHA (1990) *HIV and People with Learning Difficulties (1990)* Report of a Conference held by the South East Thames Regional Health Authority. Tunbridge Wells: SETRHA.

Tannahill, A. (1985) *What is health promotion?* Health Education Journal, 44 (4), p.167-168.

Tones, B. (1981) *Health education: Prevention or subversion?* Journal of the Royal Society of Health, (3), p.114-117

Before moving to New Zealand, James Nichol was Senior Health Promotion Adviser for Health First (formally South East London Health Promotion Service). He has undertaken staff training in HIV and learning disability and has been instumental in securing a series of local initiatives in HIV prevention and safer sex education. James was a member of the group which developed 'My Choice - My Own Choice', the safer sex educational video for people with learning disabilities.

Chapter 4

A Provider Perspective

by Simon Davies

The Story

This case study is fictional only in as much as it has been constructed by drawing on a number of real life events experienced during my work with people with learning disabilities in a number of situations and service contexts. The story is used as a vehicle to help convey an important message and is about the sequence of events in the life of one young man and the provider organisation which supports him. Although the message is for everyone, it is especially aimed at managers and support workers in all provider organisations who are working with people with learning disabilities. People with learning disabilities are one of the most disadvantaged and abused group of people in society today, being discriminated against in a variety of direct and indirect ways. The message is simple: we all have a choice. Through all our actions we can affect positive changes in society and through the actions of the people who work in services we can make very real and immediate differences to people's status and quality of life. Society has the choice to accept people with learning disabilities as true equals or by inaction, to support their continuing oppression. Through this story I hope that other provider organisations will come to recognise the challenges, to understand what action is needed and, most importantly of all, to affect positive, significant and meaningful changes in people's lives.

The Beginning

The story unfolds in an inner city borough with a diverse mix of cultures, religions and economic class, overlying vibrant and colourful communities, with deprivation, affluence, industry, commerce and unemployment all represented; in many ways typical of the contrasts and social polarisation typical of urban life in Britain today.

In this borough a young and growing organisation struggled to provide a range of residential and support services to people with learning disabilities who, in the main, had suffered appalling abuse throughout most of their lives in the back wards of inhumane environments which were both congregate and institutionalised. The organisation took some pride in the fact that it was at the leading edge of new developments: not only providing supported accommodation in small groups but also helping people to move on to further and greater independence in small flats with individual support. Whatever the aspirations of the people the organisation supported, strenuous efforts were made to see them fulfilled.

As part of these efforts the organisation took an active interest in the area of relationships, sexuality and sexual health for the people it supported. Managers and support workers understood how complex an area this was, not only from the perspective of people with learning disabilities who had experienced so much oppression, but also because of a confused and back-ward looking legal system which encourages a societal view of *dis*-ability as weakness and provides disincentives to sexual equality and expression.

This organisation has always supported, educated and trained staff, encouraging them to put the rights and wants of the people they worked with at the forefront of their thinking and action. This extended to developing and promoting audio-visual educational materials (SELHPS, 1992) and took part in extensive and innovative research (Cambridge, 1996), so a commitment to affect radical change was reflected in the production and utilisation of valued interventions in sex and safer sex education and co-operation in highlighting newly identified needs to commissioners of services for people with learning disabilities.

Challenges in Sonny's Life

The organisation was effectively 'right on' and radical in its work with service users and wider activities such as lobbying in relation to sexuality and sexual health, but this political and practical correctness was seriously challenged by an unexpected turn of events. Sonny, a young looking, forty year old man of Afro-Caribbean ethnic origin had spent thirty five of those years in the confines of a claustrophobic and dangerous 'bin' which held, at times, over one thousand 'inmates' in appallingly undignified conditions.

Five years ago he had been moved from there to his current home, sharing with four others who had not been his friends but, luckily for him, had become so. It had taken him a while to find his feet in this strange new life but he knew now the bare bones of what it meant to be more independent.

He liked the taste of it and he wanted more. Sonny liked to dress well in good quality jeans and shirts with colourful braces. He used to tell his keyworker that he liked to oil his hair and see it shine.

He attended a special class at a local college on two days a week and eventually he made it there on his own - either a short bus ride or a longer walk - unaided by support workers. Staff had helped him a lot and he appreciated that, but now he wanted more freedom to explore his widening horizons. He wanted his own flat and he was getting the staff to help him sort this out. Staff were enthusiastic and pushed their manager to find ways of supporting and resourcing this initiative. They wanted to see Sonny succeed and were impatient of bureaucratic delays.

Suddenly, over a period of just a few days, things began to change. Sonny started coming back to the house later than usual on college days and was out on other days for long periods of time. This would not normally have worried staff, but Sonny would not volunteer where he had been and sometimes appeared rather harassed and distressed when he got back. This was unlike him. Staff became further concerned when Sonny became increasingly withdrawn and refused meals, as this often indicated that he was under some sort of stress.

One day a member of staff who was off duty was taking a leisurely stroll through the local park in the early evening. She spotted Sonny standing outside a public toilet and, waving her usual greeting to him, went over to have a quick chat. As she approached, Sonny became visibly anxious, breaking into a sweat and stumbling over his words. The member of staff got a clear impression that Sonny was trying to cover something up. She began to put two and two together and felt a great sympathy for Sonny's unease. She made what turned out to be a perfect judgement, setting the pattern for the organisation's response. Polite goodbyes were said and the member of staff retreated. Sonny had been shown the respect that he had a right to expect. The incident was of course reported and the worker's hunch that Sonny was meeting men for sex was relayed. As with many such issues, senior managers were soon concerned and involved. Staff within the service were anxious but committed to supporting Sonny even though they were confused and unsure about what to do.

Challenges to the Service

The organisation was faced with a number of burning questions, some of which knocked holes in our existing policies and procedures, namely

What was *actually* happening?
What did Sonny want?
What was the risk to Sonny?
What was the organisation's legal position?
Should Sonny's movements be restricted for his own safety?
What help did Sonny need?
What advice and support did staff need?

The first and indeed only decision that was made in the 24 hours that followed was that whatever else transpired, Sonny must be helped to trust staff. A non-judgemental approach was adopted regardless of anyone's personal feelings. It must be understood that at this stage the danger of driving Sonny's activities further underground could have proved disastrous in the longer term. Sonny was to be given unconditional support. Staff were reminded not to lose touch with first principles and to remember first and foremost that Sonny had the right to be respected. Staff began to make contact with Sonny and to gently encourage him to talk to them about his experiences, including his pleasures, fears and anxieties.

Gradually, Sonny explained that he was having sexual relationships with men in public places, usually at the park. He described how he was sometimes treated well and sometimes badly. He admitted to having unprotected receptive anal intercourse which he claimed he did not particularly enjoy. However, he had consented to it because he wanted to maintain the relationships with the men he met. Apart from staff, Sonny had no other friendships or relationships with people who did not have a learning disability. It became clear that however abusive some of these contacts may have been, Sonny valued them as something of importance to him at this time in his life.

This left the organisation with exceptionally difficult decisions to make. Decisions from professional, legal and ultimately moral perspectives.

The Organisation's Position

The first thing to acknowledge in relation to the position of the provider organisation in this predicament is that its responsibilities are confused.

Further analysis reveals potential conflicts of interest which are difficult to resolve, partly because of the weakness of the law to provide clear guidance about what constitutes a severe learning disability and who is able to give consent. The law is designed to protect people from sexual exploitation and abuse but difficulty in interpretation and practice can lead to restricting peoples' sexualities and limiting their sexual rights.

The organisation aimed to support people to gain independence and enable them to develop as individuals. This included the expression of their own sexuality. These are fundamental principles and a recognition of personal and individual rights. However, the organisation also had a responsibility to protect vulnerable individuals from abuse and exploitation, to recognise such vulnerability in the people it cares for and to ensure their basic health and safety. There was also a duty to ensure that its own actions, on behalf of those with whose care it had been entrusted, were within the law.

These are compromising dilemmas when pitched against each other and the organisation's managers found themselves exceptionally challenged by them. In Sonny's case all of these issues were neatly polarised. The assessment suggested that despite being taken advantage of on occasions, Sonny was clearly expressing his desire to build relationships and to explore his sexuality. It was evident that he was himself at risk of HIV infection and was potentially a risk to others through practising unsafe sex. Not only was the sexual activity illegal in public, but the law is also discriminatory in relation to same sex behaviours and relationships between men, so there was a further legal dimension.

In these early days the organisation concluded that the only thing that had enabled them to offer any effective support to date was the fact that Sonny trusted the staff working closely with him. It was obvious that if they had tried to restrict Sonny's movements or advised him to terminate his liaisons, the problem would only be driven underground. There would be a danger of losing forever the opportunity to support Sonny and empower him take informed choices. He might never talk openly again or volunteer information to key workers. Staff were advised to be honest about their concerns but not to pressure Sonny or to make him feel any sense of disapproval.

The organisation's managers then joined keyworkers and staff team members to analyse the risk, concluding that this needed urgent attention. Health and safety issues could not be ignored. However, restricting Sonny's movements was assessed as a greater risk to Sonny's health in the longer term. He was likely to seek these experiences elsewhere anyway and it would also make him very unhappy.

To deny his experiences would have been unacceptable, but to complicate matters, the legal position could not be ignored either. Serious thought had to be given to both Sonny's vulnerability and the position of the organisation with regard to its responsibility for his care and support. After considerable debate, senior managers and support staff were unanimous in deciding that the grey areas of the law deserved to be explored and questioned in Sonny's best interests, as it was imperative that he should be assisted to take control of his own life.

The organisation took on the responsibility of testing the unclear boundaries of the law as it relates to sex and learning disability and in so doing, staff and managers ensured that the decisions made were clearly recorded and shown to be collectively agreed in order to protect individuals. These decisions also meant supporting intensive work with Sonny to educate him about the risks involved in his sexual activity. This included helping him to learn about safer sex, negotiation techniques and exit strategies. It meant encouraging him and teaching him how to be assertive about what he did and did not want in his relationships. It meant telling him about the law and about the risks involved in his activities.

It was agreed that it was important for Sonny to receive independent counselling because there was always the potential for the organisation or any of its staff to be compromised or for there to be a conflict of interests. Additionally it was seen to be vital for Sonny to have some completely confidential support from an experienced source.

Sonny needed to understand that his health and possibly even his life were at risk through unsafe sexual behaviour. The organisation sought the support of experts in the HIV field and ensured that Sonny had professional help to both understand the implications of his sexual behaviour in relation to HIV and risk and to consider whether he wanted to have an HIV test. To date he has made a firm choice not to test.

Approach

While the majority of collective effort was properly concentrated on supporting Sonny, the organisation also had to give consideration to the level and style of support needed by the staff team and managers who were closely involved. They experienced a range of difficulties. At times there were differences of opinion between them regarding the best approach to adopt, guilt about the potential risks Sonny was taking, coping with their natural instincts to protect him and feeling angry towards potential abusers.

Staff training and support sessions were organised. Personal supervision was stepped up and staff were encouraged to talk openly about their uncertainties and more importantly, about any criticisms of the direction that was being pursued. A culture was created whereby staff were supported and protected in expressing their feelings, even if they seemed outrageous or to be an over-reaction. Staff were listened to and their opinions were respected even if their views could not always be supported. This approach proved increasingly successful as it helped to unify staff in their work with Sonny. The work continued in this vein over a period of months.

Sonny continued his liaisons and, through a couple of them, participated in some gay social events which significantly increased his self esteem. He continued to talk regularly to staff and to be open about his experiences, although he rightly used his counselling sessions to talk about intimate details and feelings. Staff also learnt when Sonny was upset and he would often come to them for help. An openness developed.

Over time the education was successful and staff could tell that Sonny was practising safe sex more and more frequently. He also became more assertive about what he wanted and expected in his relationships and understood much better the need for safety. Staff tried to encourage Sonny to bring his friends home but group living is not a conducive environment and it would clearly have been an unnatural situation for him and them. Privacy was not easy to achieve and staff presence was always prohibitive. The need for greater independence for Sonny therefore became imperative. The efforts to find a flat for him intensified and plans have since become a reality. Sonny will continue to need staff support because several of his social skills are still limited but moving him to his own flat provided him with a more tailored service. His support now more accurately meets his needs and puts him more in control when staff are around to help him. More choice means more personal power.

On Reflection

Staff knew that Sonny was still at risk and they also knew that he could already be HIV positive. But Sonny knew this too and had a clearer understanding of what this meant. Even if Sonny one day gets ill with AIDS, staff and the managers involved are clear that they will not regret the actions they have taken. Sonny had a right to develop his own sexuality in his own way and to expect support from the organisation and its staff to help him to do so.

It was the responsibility of the service providers to adapt their services to meet the challenges in Sonny's life and not to enforce conformity to meet either the organisation's convenience or the unequal standards of an unjust society. This puts service providers at the cutting edge of this work and quite often they are working under a number of restrictions: legal, professional, societal and environmental. It is the responsibility of service providers to ensure that they show a responsible attitude to these complex issues on behalf of service users. The complications are challenging and stressful but not necessarily insurmountable.

Getting attitudes right from the start is essential. The following actions help:

- give respect

- show commitment

- be non-judgmental

- be honest

- give unconditional support

- don't lose touch with first principles

Staff action to a large extent affects outcomes, therefore it is important not to underestimate the power that an organisation and its staff hold. The organisation found certain actions particularly effective in this situation and these can be presented as lessons:

- create a trusting environment

- aim to hand over power

- don't deny the experiences of individuals

- be prepared to challenge unclear boundaries
- support informed choice
- educate
- analyse and assess risks and be prepared to take some
- seek appropriate and independent counselling services
- enlist professional support from specialist organisations. Help them to help the individual because they may not have the experience to do this on their own
- provide staff with quality support
- listen to what staff have to say
- provide staff with training
- and above all, be courageous

Some of the above, such as planning with staff and staff training can be done proactively. Service providers do not need to wait for a crisis in order to act. Reflecting on the outcomes for Sonny of the approach adopted by the organisation, we can see that he benefited in several ways:

- gaining self esteem
- finding openness in those who supported him, generating a trusting environment
- feeling safe
- developing independence
- improving knowledge and understanding
- learning about rights
- making choices
- gaining power

It would of course be inappropriate to conclude a chapter about service providers without mentioning resources. It does not necessarily take much but it does take some money, effort and time. Service providers should organise some flexible financial resources which can be deployed quickly and at short notice if necessary, in order to pay for such things as counselling or educational materials.

Work may need to be done to free up managers, time in order to support staff and work more closely with them in the early stages. Service providers should also develop networks of specialist support. These will prove invaluable.

It is important to challenge local commissioners of services to address these issues themselves and support to service providers in order that they recognise the dilemmas facing providers and the need for more funds and resources. In particular make them aware of the legal grey areas.

These are changing times and providers have got to adapt to meet the challenge of changing needs. HIV is with us in this society but so are the rights of people with learning disabilities to develop their own sexuality, and the rights of people with HIV and AIDS. Service providers must meet the issues head on and not ignore them. Finding positive ways of tackling the sorts of conflict that have been described here must be our priority for the future. We do have a choice about the positions we take on these issues and we still hold a lot of power over the lives of people with learning disabilities. We must use that power responsibly and in the best interests of people with learning disabilities.

References

Cambridge, P. (1996)   *Men with learning disabilities who have sex with men in public places: mapping the needs of services and users in south east London.* Journal of Intellectual Disability Research. Vol.40, No.3.

SELPHS (1992)   *My Choice, My Own Choice* (video), Pavilion Publishing Brighton.

Simon Davies is Director of Southside Partnership, a provider of housing and staff support services for people with learning disabilities and people with mental health needs in South London. He leads the empower sexuality advisory group in Lambeth which works in the area of learning disability, and was a member of the group which developed 'My Choice - My Own Choice', the safer sex educational video for people with leaning disabilities.

Chapter 5

Safer Sex Work With Men With Learning Disabilities Who Have Sex With Men

by David Thompson

It would have helped if we had started with a better understanding of how sex with men was experienced by men with learning disabilities when AIDS arrived. Instead, services had chosen to remain ignorant. The only experts were the men with learning disabilities themselves and they had never been asked what the sex they had was like. Instead they had been told off, told not to and told to find a girlfriend. This largely remains the starting point for work aspiring to protect men with learning disabilities. In this chapter I describe the work I have undertaken as part of the Sex Education Team at Horizon NHS Trust as a guide to others undertaking safer sex work and to influence those with responsibility for the sexual health of people with learning disabilities.

Priorities

As a gay man living in the community which has borne the brunt of the AIDS epidemic in this country, it is clear to me that the needs of men who have sex with men should take priority in any HIV initiative. Despite the monthly HIV and AIDS figures which consistently show that men who have sex with men are the most affected group, those charged with responsibility for prevention have been slow to take this on board. Trying to prioritise this group in learning disabilities is particularly difficult because of their invisibility and the secrecy which surrounds their behaviour.

Men with learning disabilities essentially have sex in three main contexts. The first is with other men with learning disabilities who share the same service. The second is with men who do not have learning disabilities but with whom they have an ongoing relationship. This relationship may be based on friendship or the abuse of a family or professional role. The third is accessing public toilets and other locations where men meet for sex. Although HIV infection is possible in each of these contexts, specific attention will be given

71

here to the last, the priority suggested by the epidemiology of HIV. Risk of exposure to the HIV virus increases with the number of partners and sexual contacts. This priority reflects known cases of HIV amongst men with learning disabilities (Brown, 1991; Dent, Vergnaud & Piachaud, 1994).

There is only localised evidence about the prevalence of men with learning disabilities seeking sex with men in public toilets (Cambridge, 1996). Amongst male referrals to the Sex Education Team it was found that one third were involved in cottaging. Because of the independence skills necessary to travel to public toilets unaccompanied there is a bias towards more able men. Such a high figure is particularly remarkable when it is noted that there was no mention of such sexual activity in the literature before the nineties and suggests that many services have for a long time, ignored the issues it presents rather than seeking to ensure professional support.

My own research and the work of colleagues has identified some common features in the experiences of men with learning disabilities who cottage, which are of value for informing safer sex work. The most significant is the usual passivity of men with learning disabilities in their sexual encounters. Typically, men with learning disabilities wait for someone to approach them and simply comply with their sexual demands. This is most acutely identified by men's accounts of almost exclusively being penetrated when anal sex takes place, when this is neither their choice nor preference. This was described almost unanimously as being painful (it does not have to be with a sensitive partner and a lubricant). It is also important to understand that the men with learning disabilities visit public toilets for more complex reasons than simply seeking sexual pleasure, including providing an exciting way of passing empty time, an opportunity to make contact with men who do not have learning disabilities, or possibly gaining some small financial reward. These features are more fully detailed elsewhere (Thompson, 1994).

Some workers feel particularly troubled by the legality of sex in public toilets and feel obliged to instruct the men not to cottage. Such a response will not facilitate communication in safer sex work with men who cottage. In practice, many police forces recognise that there are more pressing demands on their time than worrying about what consenting adults are doing. Even when arrests are made, good legal advice can successfully avoid prosecution. Where men with learning disabilities have been found hanging around public toilets, charges have not been brought because of the identified learning disability.

My own advice to men with learning disabilities is to watch out for the police and leave if they see them.

Methods

There are different options for providing safer sex work with men with learning disabilities who have sex with men, including individual work and group work. I suggest individual work offers the best opportunity to support the men's needs. Although group work does have the attraction of peer support it must be recognised that this support is not necessarily forthcoming when the subject is sex between men. I have worked in men's groups where over half of the participants have had sex with men but were unable to make these truly safe spaces to talk about sex with men because of the homophobia of group members (not least amongst those with such experience). As yet, no group exclusively for men who have had sex with men has been run by the team. Now in the process of setting up such a group, I am aware that all the participants are very likely to need some preparatory individual attention. Minimally, this would help them acknowledge that a place in a group for men who have sex with men was appropriate for them, thereby avoiding the possibility that they will enter the group and deny their behaviour.

Who should do the work?

The debate as to whether the man should already know the worker or have independent specialist help is important but hypothetical in most situations where specialists are unavailable. Even where specialist support is possible, input is likely to be short term, and there remains a need for someone to have a long term commitment to the man. The skills required of the worker are the ability to communicate sensitively with people with learning disabilities (a skill safer sex specialists outside learning disability are likely to lack), an unprejudiced understanding of sex between men and some confidence to discuss sexual matters.

This skill list does not demand that the worker is a gay man. There are many other people, usually women, who have the necessary qualities. Gay men do have the advantage of being able to share experiences of sex with men, but not all gay men have the political subtlety or professional sensitivity to distinguish between the wider gay agenda and the specific needs of men with learning disabilities who have sex with men.[1]

---

1.   See the debate between MacManus, Bainbridge & Thompson in Health Psychology Update, Issue 21, September 1995 for an example of this tension.

Within both the fields of learning disability and HIV prevention, peer approaches to work have gained popularity. This model does not necessarily transfer well to targeted prevention work with men with learning disabilities who have sex with men, largely because there are few men with learning disabilities who hold positive attitudes about sex with men. There also needs to be caution about peer ability to fulfil the other criteria above and to ensure the response is in the man's best interests.

If the work is to proceed on a one-to-one basis it is important to address safeguards for both the worker and the man with learning disabilities. For the worker, safeguards include prior management support for the work high enough to defend criticism. It is in both people's interest for the service to agree a location for the work which strikes a balance between space which ensuring total privacy and yet is close to other staff. Any policies for staff working alone with clients should be adhered to.

Acknowledgement

Poor self-esteem with regard to having sex with men is known to be a predictor of unsafe sex. It can be argued that the ability of men to acknowledge experiences is some measure of their self-esteem. Specific knowledge of the men's experiences can also clarify the task for the worker in providing crucial information about the context and environment in which unsafe sex may occur. For these reasons I have always felt it important to enable the men to talk about some of their experiences. This task is very demanding. Even when men have been witnessed having sex with men the level of denial can be enormous. A pattern is discernible, in that the more able the man, the more he is aware of society's disapproval of homosexuality and so the more inhibited he is to disclosure.

For a man with learning disabilities to disclose sexual contact with men he must first be confident of not receiving a negative reaction. This places responsibility on the worker to convince him that this will not be the case. In practice, it means continually providing a positive message about sex between men. The worker must demonstrate that he believes sex between men is good. It might be enough just to say so. This was the case with one man who offered that he had had sex with men during an introductory meeting, much to the surprise of the keyworker in the room who thought they knew him. Good resources provide powerful support for this message. A lot is said implicitly if the workers are confident in their use of images depicting two men having sex. The line drawings in *Sex and the Three R's* have proved invaluable for this work. The video *Piece by Piece* has also been useful in providing a catalyst for other men to begin to speak about their experiences.

Identifying as gay, I have always been of the option that it is appropriate for me to reinforce the central message by telling men with learning disabilities that I have sex with men. I do not believe that this should be any more an issue than people with learning disabilities knowing whether staff are married or have children. Those who feel that lesbian and gay staff should not *come out* to their clients, need to take responsibility for the painful isolation felt by men with learning disabilities who commonly know no other men who have sex with men. It is often the case that even in organisations where some staff feel confident enough to come out to their colleagues, they feel a need to censor this with their clients.

My disclosure to men with learning disabilities may help them to understand that it is not only them, nor just other men with learning disabilities who have sex with men, but that it is also the case for some men who they perceive as powerful. It has a similar effect to me telling men that I masturbate. They are forced to review their perceptions about staff and can make connections between their experience and those of other people. Without hesitation, I tell men that I play with myself since, as the vast majority of men do so, it is no more revealing than telling them that I have a leg. There is more at stake telling them that I have sex with men. Caution is necessary because other people with power in the men's life may not appreciate the value of this strategy. If they learn about it they may attempt to sabotage the work. Potentially, the men may misunderstand the disclosure as an invitation for sex. In one situation where this happened, the man experienced painful rejection when I explained why this was not going to happen. In practice, I choose not to give the men specific details about the context of my sexual experiences with men. This is because in common with most staff, my life opportunities bear little resemblance to those of the men with whom I work.

The above techniques, sharing experience and attitudes, using explicit resources and personal disclosure may have to be repeated week after week before men have the confidence to talk about their own experiences. With one man this took over two years, even though it was widely understood by staff that he had sex with men. Many men will stay silent as the positive messages they may hear during individual work fail to counter accumulated

75

homophobic influences. Some men will not disclose because they are afraid of what will happen to the information and who the worker may tell. Attention is given below to the complexity of confidentiality.

Power, Consent and Abuse

As important as the men knowing that sex between men can be good is an understanding of when it is not good. This is a difficult balance to achieve. Some specialist resources seem only able to cope with depicting images of abuse (e.g. Life Horizon slides). Conversely, there are examples of gay positive work appearing blind to the possibility of power exploitation between men (e.g. McLeod, unpubl.). The message is more complex than 'sex between men is good if they both want it' but this is a useful beginning. Images of both consented and unconsented intimate contact between men can help to emphasise this point. Typically, men with learning disabilities who have been abused by men will feel guilty about what has happened to them therefore it is important to identify that it is the abuser and not the abused who did something wrong.

The men should also know that sex with staff and sex between adults and children is wrong and the abuser in such situations should again be identified. The age of consent for sex between men is moving toward equality with that for heterosexual sex therefore there is little point in wasting valuable time on this discriminatory detail. Other legislation leads to uncertainty about severe learning disability and who it is illegal to have sex with. It is very unlikely that men with learning disabilities who cottage would be covered by this legislation because they demonstrate considerable ability in being able to move independently in the community. However, they still need to be warned against having sex with women or men who are significantly less able.

Only a small proportion of the sexual experiences with men would be defined by law as abusive, although in the vast majority of cases there is likely to be an abuse of power, namely one man getting his sexual desires met at the expense of the other. This is most evident from the familiar experience of men with learning disabilities who, cottage of being penetrated when anal sex takes place. It is not their choice and they are unable to explain why it happens that way round. However, the balance of power can tip in their favour if they are having sex with other people with learning disabilities, particularly women and less able men. Supporting men in situations with an uneven distribution of power involves encouraging them not to do anything they or their partners do not want, and helping them to gain some insight into who is not being 'fair'.

The line between power differences in relation to sexual abuse is difficult to draw and its thickness is subject to interpretation. It is very difficult for a worker to whom a disclosure of abuse or a negative experience of sex is made to decide whether they should seek to empower the man in their relationship or take action to stop it. An awareness is required of the very ambivalent feelings the man is likely to have about sex with men. There will be guilt about having sex with men, overlapped by potential excitement, pleasure and painful experiences of anal sex. Care should be taken to wait before making assumptions about what a man's real experience has been. It is, after all, easier for a man to say he did not want to have the sex than to admit to enjoying sex with men.

Giving men with learning disabilities permission to talk about sex with men also gives some men the voice to disclose instances of sexual abuse. Workers should obviously provide support if this is the case. In doing so, they will need to guard against simplistic and homophobic assumptions suggesting that the experience has made them homosexual or that it is proof that they really do not want sex with men.

Identity

For any man with learning disabilities who is able to acknowledge a desire to have sex with men, the question of sexual identity arises. This is a matter of choice for the man concerned. An identity should not be imposed on him nor should the choice be forced. There are many good reasons why a man with learning disabilities who has sex with men will resist taking on a gay identity. For a start, it may have little meaning for him apart from associating it with a term of abuse. Further, it is a brave man who says that he is gay and so much harder if you do not know any other gay men. It is worthwhile ensuring that the man knows that some men who have sex with men say they are gay (many do not; most of the men who have sex in public toilets are married or live with women and have straight identities). Similar caution is required if the man has sex with both women and men with regard to a bisexual identity. Unfortunately, many workers fail to understand the difference between sexual activity and sexual identity, believing that the former determines the latter and so label their clients accordingly. Gay positive workers should consider the very different lives of men with learning disabilities who have sex with

77

men compared with gay identified men, and question the relevance of a gay identity for many men with learning disabilities.

If men start to explore taking on a gay identity for themselves, it can be very empowering and lead to their integration into elements of the gay community. If this is done, consideration should be given to how the man would likely be received in a non-learning disability setting and what the man's own expectations are.

Information

This is the most straightforward part of the work. The aim is to ensure the man knows in what situations he is at risk and how risk can be reduced or avoided. There is a consensus among those people who work with people with learning disabilities that this information needs to be simplified. Therefore, talk is of getting AIDS rather than HIV and giving a clear warning that people who get AIDS die instead of trying to accurately describe the uncertain futures of those who are HIV positive.

Basically, the man needs to know he can get AIDS from anal sex without a condom, therefore it is very important to try to use condoms with any partner. With all but the most able men I have disregarded the risk of HIV transmission from oral sex. This is because the risk is known to be very low and it allows a clear emphasis on the activity which puts them at greatest risk. Further, there is very little usage of condoms for oral sex for any men having sex with men and therefore it would be exceptionally difficult for men with learning disabilities to get their partners to comply.

This work is effectively done by asking the man with learning disabilities how he can get AIDS, presenting him with a series of line drawings of different sexual activities. It is worthwhile asking the man to put a condom (wrapped) on the men who need to use condoms, as it may not be immediately obvious who should wear a condom when two men are having anal sex.

Skills

It is important that men with learning disabilities are familiar with handling and using condoms. A model penis to practice on is essential here and the 'deluxe' versions which feature ejaculation are very useful in trying to explain how condoms prevent infection. Asking men to try putting a condom on the model can highlight some of the problems they may have, including difficulties in opening the packet and determining which way the condom rolls down the penis. The worker should recognise that success on a static model in a session does not mean that a man would be able to put one on himself during sex. There may not be the luxuries of time, light or a penis which stays erect. It is worthwhile encouraging the men to practice putting them on while masturbating and asking them how they get on. Condoms need to be made freely available to the men. Men are often reluctant to take them home however, because of fear about what other people will say. This points to a major task for the worker in also undertaking training with other carers.

Research indicates that the greatest risk of HIV infection to men with learning disabilities is not their own failure to use condoms but that of their partners, since they are almost exclusively penetrated during sex in the situations which pose the greatest risk of HIV infection (Thompson, 1994). Greater energy therefore needs to be directed at giving the men strategies to stop partners who are trying to penetrate them without a condom than to enhancing their own skills in condom use. As much as possible, work in this priority area should reflect the reality of the sexual encounters. For example, there is rarely any conversation prior to sex in public toilets and so there should be an acknowledgement of the difficulty of breaking the silence to ask for a condom to be used.

It is worthwhile clarifying what options are available to a man with learning disabilities if he is about to be penetrated without a condom. The first is to accept the situation or to try to avert it. The latter needs to be recognised as incredibly hard, as it has been shown how men are regularly unable to challenge their partners when they are enduring painful anal sex. General assertiveness work can be of benefit here, as well as ensuring the man is clear about what is at stake if he does not take any action. If the man does find the strength to assert himself, he has the option of trying to insist that his partner uses a condom or not to have anal sex. I am ambivalent about guiding the men at this point. Ideally I would rather they rejected the anal sex because it is not something they enjoy, although it may be less demanding to negotiate condom use. If anal sex is avoided or a condom is not available, the man should know that there are still possibilities to continue the sex safely. However, he is likely to have reasonable fears that any attempt to avoid unsafe sex could terminate the sexual encounter. Role play can be employed to help this work, but can also easily be misinterpreted as an invitation for sex from the worker.

HIV Antibody Testing

Telling men with learning disabilities that unprotected anal sex puts them at risk of AIDS is not the same as saying that previous incidents may have already infected them. On rare occasions men have worked out the possibility of the second from the first, with the majority staying untroubled by their current HIV status. In these latter situations, the worker needs to decide whether to directly point out the man's current risk. This could be of benefit because it may underline that AIDS is a real risk to the man concerned. On the other hand, the man could be alarmed about having to confront the possibility of infection. In practice, men find it very hard to understand this uncertainty and largely remain apparently untroubled by their status. The difficulty of conceptualising latent infection is a factor here.

From the above it is clear that without very specific prompting men are rarely concerned about their HIV status and so are unlikely to want to confirm it through HIV antibody testing. For those few men who do appreciate their current risk, being given some information about testing may encourage them to want to take the test. Regardless of the man's position on testing, services are often keen to facilitate a test where they believe a man is at risk of HIV. This is usually without prior consideration about how they would respond to the result.

British Medical Association guidelines are clear. HIV testing should only be carried out with the informed consent of the individual concerned. To adhere to this stipulation, men with learning disabilities would have to appreciate both the medical and social implications of a positive or negative result. For example, they should be prepared for the possibility of social and service exclusion and for the possible negative reaction of carers. This demands considerable preparation for a test. A suggested model for good practice is for information about the test and an exploration of the possible consequences to be first undertaken by the worker. If the worker is satisfied of the man's continued desire to have the test and his understanding of it, he could be referred to a special clinic where the clinicians should be briefed not to proceed with a test if the man does not demonstrate an acceptable level of informed consent.

In reality, current practice often only seeks the man's agreement to a test, with the man neither requesting the test, or having an adequate knowledge of it. In such circumstances, workers should advocate for the man, pointing out that the test is proceeding contrary to law. Recognising that many men with learning disabilities are unable to give valid consent to an HIV test does not necessarily deny their access to it. As with any medical procedure, it may be legally undertaken on a person unable to consent if it can be demonstrated that it is in their best interests. The 'best interests' criteria could possibly be satisfied by access to prophylactic treatments.

Special Clinics

Exploration of the possibility of an HIV test may lead to a visit to a clinic which specialises in sexually transmitted diseases. There are however also other reasons why attending such a clinic would be useful. If it is known that a man has frequent intimate sexual contact with many men there is a significant risk of contracting sexual diseases other than HIV. In addition to times when there might be symptoms, regular visits (6 months - 1 year) will help minimise the effect of any infection. Clinics can also provide hepatitis B vaccination which should be arranged for any man who cottages.

Apart from being embarrassing places to visit, the experience can be very confusing because of the different roles of staff. Commonly, a first visit will entail giving details to the receptionist, a consultation with a doctor, specimens taken by a nurse and safer sex advice from a health advisor. Ideally, men should be prepared for this and be warned about where the specimens will be taken from. Prior contact with the clinic is useful to clarify that the man will have special needs and to negotiate the role for the workers, including their possible access to confidential information concerning the man.

Confidentiality

Confidentiality with a man with learning disabilities may be of benefit in fostering trust between him and the worker. The knowledge that specific information will not be passed on to anyone else in the service may make a difference over what he is prepared to disclose. Further, knowing that he has control over what information is to be passed on could be experienced as empowering: a key aim of safer sex work. Together, these present a powerful argument for offering men with learning disabilities a confidential service. Some policies of organisations do not allow this. Further, absolute confidentiality is never possible because of the specific requirements

81

of the Children Act (1989) which insist that all professionals pass on information where harm to a child is disclosed. This is not the place to debate the merits of confidentiality relating to sexual abuse, although there are some specific considerations relating to HIV risk which should be considered.

A typical scenario in my experience, is a man who discloses that he cottages as an unexpected consequence of individual work on another sexual matter. The details show that he is putting himself at significant risk of HIV. Work proceeds which tries to give him the skills to avoid unsafe sex but it becomes apparent that his passivity and inassertiveness mean that he is unlikely to be able to put this into practice, even if the input is sustained over many months. To choose not to inform the man's wider service of this situation amounts to giving the man total responsibility for his own protection when he has demonstrated an inability to hold that responsibility. Talking to the service allows other workers to take some responsibility for his protection (through extending his choice of activities or increased supervision). Even men who reveal some potential to protect themselves from HIV are likely to require ongoing support which would be very difficult to guarantee without communicating his future needs to the service.

For these reasons, I have occasionally gone against a man's wishes and informed the service of the man's activities. This is not easily done but the alternative of holding on to information and responsibility for his protection, is much less attractive. Clearly, this has implications for what is said about confidentiality. In practice I tend to be very guarded about suggesting that I can, as a worker within a wider service context, maintain complete confidentiality.

Evaluation

The scenario depicted above, of a man with learning disabilities lacking the skills to prevent unsafe sex with men after specialist safer sex input is typical and others have not acknowledged this. It might be suggested that other workers are simply more effective but there is little evidence of this since the cumulative experience of the Sex Education Team is probably the greatest available anywhere. There is currently no standardised assessment available to measure a man with learning disabilities' ability to avoid unsafe sex. Box 1 below, highlights what are likely to be key indicators.

BOX I
KEY INDICATORS FOR ASSESSING ABILITY TO AVOID UNSAFE SEX

Knowledge
Knowing how AIDS (HIV) is transmitted and treated

Motivation
Believing that AIDS (and by implication HIV) could affect them

Self-esteem
Caring enough about themselves to want to avoid unsafe sex

Skills
Having strategies available to avoid unsafe sex

Condoms
Having easy access to condoms and lubricants

Assertiveness
Having the confidence to put the strategies into place

Knowledge, skills and condoms are relatively straight forward to provide and assess. Much more difficult is the enhancement and measurement of motivation, self-esteem and assertiveness. These are all related to the marginalisation of people with learning disabilities and so are perhaps unrealistic goals for individual work which can do little to change inequalities in society.

One way of evaluating work is to stay in contact with the man and listen to what is happening in his sexual contacts. It is important to recognise how men are likely to try to please the worker by saying they are using condoms. Acquiescence can be avoided by ensuring the worker indicates how very difficult it is to avoid unsafe sex.

Working intimately with men with learning disabilities on safer sex has exposed me and my colleagues to some very upsetting aspects of sexual contact

83

between men. Let me be clear that it is not sex between men, anal sex, the location of the sex in public toilets nor the lack of an established relationship which is of concern. The problem is the exploitation of power by men without learning disabilities which renders men with learning disabilities vulnerable to painful sexual experiences and HIV infection. This gendered power is equally found in sex within marriages and in men with learning disabilities' own relationships with women, as Michelle McCarthy's chapter demonstrates. It is important to recognise that there is no contradiction addressing this abuse of power and taking a gay positive stance in work with men with learning disabilities who cottage. Indeed, to do otherwise would return many men with learning disabilities to silence or fail to equip them with the skill they need to protect themselves.

References

Brown, D. (1991).   *HIV Infection in Persons With Prior Mental Retardation*, AIDS Care, 3, 2 165-173.

Dent, J., Vergnaud, *HIV Infection and People With Learning Disabilities*. The
S. & Piachaud, J.   Lancet, 343, 919.
(1994)

McLeod, J.   *More Than One Barrier: HIV & AIDS and Men With*
(unpubl.).   *Intellectual Disabilities Who Have Sex With Men: An Educational Needs Assessment*, Melbourne Victoria AIDS Council.

Thompson, D.J.   *The Sexual Experiences of Men With Learning Disabilities*
(1994).   *Having Sex With Men: Issues for HIV Prevention. Sexuality & Disability*, Human Sciences, New York, 12, 221-242.

David Thompson works jointly as Research Fellow at the Tizard Centre and as Team Leader of The Sex Education Team at Harperbury, providing a specialist sexuality service to people with learning disabilities and staff. His work interests have focused on men with learning disabilities who have sex with men and he is currently undertaking research with Hilary Brown on men with learning disabilities who sexually abuse or have unacceptable behaviours.

Chapter 6

HIV and Heterosexual Sex

by Michelle McCarthy

Background to My Work

This chapter concentrates on some of the practical aspects of doing HIV prevention work with people with learning disabilities in the context of heterosexual sex. This covers the majority of my own experience from work in the Sex Education Team (1989 - 1993) at Harperbury. In recent years I have continued to do a limited amount of work there as well as in other services as a result of my current work base at the Tizard Centre, University of Kent.

My own direct experience is exclusively of working with women with learning disabilities. All that I have learnt about sexuality and safer sex work with men with learning disabilities has stemmed from the women I have worked with and my male colleagues on the Sex Education Team. At the time of writing this chapter, my colleagues and I had collectively accumulated experience of working with about 70 women and 140 men on an individual basis. We did not undertake in-depth safer sex work with every person, but with a significant proportion.

General Observations

Before discussing the key lessons from my safer sex work with women, it is appropriate to consider some general points regarding HIV prevention work with people with learning disabilities. As a team, we have always made a distinction between two primary inputs, namely giving people *general information* about HIV, which we hoped would prove directly useful or simply expand people's knowledge base, and making a genuine and concerted effort to achieve some *specific behaviour* change, enabling people to get to a point where they could regularly practice safer sex. We always felt that the former could be done in a group, but the latter needed to be done on an individual basis. All our work has been done on a single sex basis: this gives the person with learning disabilities the maximum chance of identifying with their safer sex advisor and feeling comfortable about asking questions. It can if appropriate, also offer an opportunity to look at shared life experiences and shared success or difficulty in achieving safer sexual practices (McCarthy, 1994).

Before doing safer sex work with people with learning disabilities, it is necessary to try to get across some basic information about what AIDS is, why they do not want to get it and how not to get it. Although this is stating the obvious, it is worth stating because it is very difficult to do. For many people with learning disabilities, the distinction between HIV and AIDS is simply too complicated. From one angle, it is not strictly necessary information. To protect yourself, you don't need to know about viruses and the immune system, merely how the infection can be transmitted. Some HIV educators and education materials do not emphasise the difference between the two (Young Adult Institute, 1987 & McCarthy and Thompson, 1994), although others do (People First, undated; O'Sullivan & Gillies, 1993). It is my contention that in working with people whose understanding and concentration is limited, it is helpful to prioritise and simplify information. Sacrificing accuracy for the sake of getting the message across is sometimes necessary (Jacobs et al., 1989). We choose to talk about AIDS rather than HIV, even though this is not accurate, because many people with learning disabilities have already heard about AIDS, which gives us something to build on.

The practical skills required to obtain and use condoms should not be underestimated. For example, many people with learning disabilities find it extremely difficult to open the small foil packet. By far the most difficult thing for most people is understanding that the condom only rolls one way and to turn it over if it does not roll freely. Many people with learning disabilities simply pull it until it is rips or give up trying, saying 'it doesn't work'. Despite having been shown many times and despite much practice, the procedure of turning it over remains very difficult to understand and carry out for many people. These kinds of difficulties argue for a practical, hands-on teaching approach, whereby individuals get a chance to practice on a model penis, not merely relying on people learning from looking at a leaflet or video (Rees & Berchert, 1992).

Another general point to remember in doing safer sex work with both women and men with learning disabilities is not to always take people's initial response at face value. This is not to suggest that people with learning disabilities routinely lie about sexual matters, but just like everyone else they usually want to please, to give the right answers and to be thought well of. When it comes to safer sex and condom use it is easy to work out the right answers. In my own experience, many women with learning disabilities will say they use condoms when the subject is first introduced, yet when it comes to handling them in sex education sessions it becomes quite apparent that they have never seen one before and have no idea how to use them. It is similarly wise to be cautious with men with learning disabilities who say after their first lesson that they are regularly using condoms for sex. The Sex Education Team's experience is that this is not usually the case. Once again, this should not be viewed as a deliberate attempt to deceive, but the men too will probably want to please by giving the right response.

Working with couples sometimes produces conflicting accounts, as the example of Susan and Donald shows (nb. names have been changed to respect confidentiality). Both were given safer sex advice and condoms. Donald maintained throughout his sex education sessions that he was regularly using condoms when he had sex with Susan, but Susan, in her sex education sessions, was adamant that he did not use them. As they could not both be giving a true account, we had to decide what motivation each might have for saying something that was not true and continued to reinforce the safer sex messages with both.

Some unexpected issues can arise when introducing and giving condoms to people. Francesca asked for vast numbers of condoms to be given to her during sex education sessions, although she was unable to say why she wanted so many. Each week she would ask for more and more, although at the same time she was not able or willing to give any indication of the success or otherwise she was having in negotiating their use with her sexual partners. It later transpired (through a conversation with her key worker) that Francesca was in fact hoarding them in her room and not using them at all. For people who have few personal possessions and little access to material goods, being given things can be meaningful and they may well not want to part with them. It took some time for Francesca to believe that the supply of condoms was not going to stop and that she had no need to hoard them and for her to understand that condoms had no inherent value in themselves (other than to protect her and her sexual partners).

One of the most important things to consider is that in most learning disability services (community and hospital based) and in many family homes, people with learning disabilities are given no access to private and dignified spaces appropriate for having sex in. Even where people with learning disabilities have their own bedrooms, they often feel that it is not allowed to have a sexual partner in them. In many services there are rules against this, but even where there are not, strong social and psychological barriers may still exist. Many people with learning disabilities are consequently obliged to take sexual opportunities as and where they arise and both men and women can clearly explain that their sexual encounters are almost always very rushed (McCarthy & Thompson, 1993). This is not an environment which is in any way conducive to having safer let alone pleasurable sex and such factors are beyond the control of individual people with learning disabilities. It is the responsibility of service providers to attend to such issues.

Moving on to the more detailed area of safer sex education, it is necessary to appreciate the dynamics of the actual sexual encounters between men and women with learning disabilities. If I had to sum up our conclusions succinctly about heterosexual safer sex work, I would make the following key point. Generally speaking, women with learning disabilities have the motivation to have safer sex, but not the power to make it happen and men with learning disabilities have the power, but not the motivation. The rest of this chapter attempts to explain this observation, which is regarded by some as very contentious. In addition, I will suggest some ways services can move forward with these issues.

Working with Women with Learning Disabilities
Before doing safer sex work in detail, it is important to try to build up a picture of precisely the kind of sex the woman is having, including the sexual activities she engages in and with whom. This is obviously working on a very personal level and women should never be questioned about this for the sake of it. I believe it is essential to know the context of people's sexual activity in order to be able to respond appropriately. A very obvious point is to find out if the woman is having penetrative sex, because if she is not then there is no problem with HIV.

Sex between men and women with learning disabilities almost always involves penetrative sex, most always vaginal and often anal (McCarthy, 1993), but it is important to check. It is helpful to know whether the sex takes place in the context of an established relationship, based on affection or love, or whether the contact is primarily or purely sexual, as this will also inform the rest of the work (McCarthy, 1994).

To find out what kind of sex women are having, it can be helpful to use explicit line drawings, such as those found in numerous specialist sex education packs (McCarthy & Thompson, 1993; O'Sullivan & Gillies, 1993). The reason for using such visual images is that they can help people talk about things that are otherwise embarrassing or difficult. Few women are comfortable or confident enough about their sexuality to sit and simply reel off a list of sexual things they do. Many would anyway not possess the vocabulary to do so. In my experience the majority of women with learning disabilities are not overly embarrassed to say which sexual activities they engage in, although occasionally there may be embarrassment if I mention sexual activities they do not do. Neither are they usually offended by questions or statements about sex, except with regard to oral sex on a man, when women sometimes take offence at any suggestion that they might engage in this activity. I will return to this point later in the chapter, as it is a very significant consideration.

In the course of finding out from the women what they do sexually, it is not uncommon for them to ask me what kinds of sex I have. Although this is sometimes embarrassing for me, I always answer, as it seems perfectly appropriate for women to have an interest in my sexual life, when I am so obviously interested in theirs. Having said that, I find most women are in fact not *that* interested, so the information I divulge about myself is brief and only given when requested. I would not volunteer such information. Some sex educators feel it important *not* to divulge personal information about their own sexual lives, in order to maintain boundaries or protect their own confidentiality (this may be a particular concern for lesbian or gay workers in homophobic environments), but two-way sharing of information is certainly consistent with feminist research and practice (Finch, 1984; Oakley, 1981).

As indicated, it has been my experience that most women with learning disabilities do not show any resistance to practising safer sex. They usually do not need much persuading that it would be a good idea not to get any diseases or infections from sex. The only exception I have encountered was in a group setting, where two women with mild learning disabilities, Angela and Mandy, were very vocal in expressing their belief that *they* did not need to consider protection as *their* boyfriends were alright. Despite my conviction

89

that that they did need to consider protection, as Mandy had had sexually transmitted diseases in the past and Angela's boyfriend was known to be sexually active with several other men and women, both women were resistant to the idea of protection, hostile and ridiculing towards me for having raised the topic and effectively prevented the group from discussing the issue. This experience, and many other positive experiences of addressing the issue sensitively in individual work, has reinforced my belief that one-to-one work is the most appropriate way to address an individual's vulnerability and concerns.

Negotiating Skills

The great majority of women with learning disabilities show a willingness to learn about condoms and most express a desire to use them for sex. The difficulty arises in teaching and transferring negotiating skills. Negotiating safer sex between two people with learning disabilities, like any two people, is about power, namely who has it and who does not, who can ask for what they want and who cannot, who is likely to be listened to and respected and who is not.

It has been my experience that most women with learning disabilities do not exert much, if any, power in their sexual encounters with men. This also seems the case whether they are in long term committed relationships where they love their boyfriend (or even husband) or where it is purely a sexual encounter. This is reflected by the fact that the vast majority of women with learning disabilities do not get the kinds of sex they want or enjoy (McCarthy, 1993). As both men and women with learning disabilities have told us over and over again, the typical sexual encounter is a rushed affair, involving almost exclusively vaginal and/or anal penetration. When non-penetrative sex is part of the repertoire, it is almost always the woman rubbing the man's penis. Although it is important to think about and encourage non-penetrative sex as safer sexual activities, safer-sex advisors have to be aware that essentially they will be suggesting things largely outside the established pattern of sex and which may be (and I would argue *should* be) sometimes purely for the woman's sexual pleasure. This goes against the pattern of how most men and woman with learning disabilities relate sexually and raises questions about who and what sex is for. This does not imply that this should not be done, rather it acknowledges that it is actually very difficult to do. Unless advice is set in the real context of what is currently happening sexually for individuals and followed through with an evaluation of how realistic the suggestions are, it is likely to be pretty ineffective advice.

My experience has shown that it is important to be particularly aware of, and sensitive to, feelings women with learning disabilities may have regarding oral sex. By this I mean specifically a woman giving oral sex to a man. A man giving oral sex to a woman has only been within the experience of one of the 65 women with learning disabilities that I have spoken to. This says it all. Also, only one of the 65 women with learning disabilities has said anything positive about giving oral sex to a man. This was a woman whose identity was very much bound up with what she saw as her ability to give sexual pleasure to men who did not have learning disabilities. That is not to detract from the positive feelings she expressed about oral sex, but it is important to understand that consideration. All the other women I have met have expressed very strong and very negative feelings about oral sex. These are women who largely tolerate painful and upsetting anal penetration and who may submit to being used sexually by a variety of men. Yet when it comes to oral sex, they express their feelings in no uncertain terms. Quite why so many women with learning disabilities have such negative feelings about oral sex is difficult to understand and is something I am trying to find out more about in my research and ongoing work. Whether women with learning disabilities have more negative feelings than other women is also very difficult to establish, given the paucity of research on the topic. A possible explanation might be that women with learning disabilities find it difficult to say that they like oral sex, but even if this were so, due to the social prohibitions about it that still exist for some people, it does not explain why this is not the case with anal sex, which if anything is associated with more social prohibitions.

Given the fact that the vast majority of women with learning disabilities I have met have said that they strongly dislike oral sex, I have seen little point in presenting it to women as a safer sex alternative. I would also advise caution about presenting it as such to men with learning disabilities who have sex with women, as the chances of them finding a woman who would enjoy engaging in that activity are slim.

To summarise my observations on safer sex work with women with learning disabilities, I think they need the following inputs from sex educators to help ensure successful work:

*   self-esteem work to help think of themselves as people worth looking after and as people who could do these things

- a reasonable understanding of the issues associated with AIDS, what HIV or AIDS is, and why they or their partners don't want to get it

- reasonable communication skills, probably verbally, but if not, very good non-verbal skills to enable them to communicate with others

- sexual partners who also have a reasonable understanding of the issues, who also communicate, who respect and who will listen and take notice of what they say

- a realisation that their role in sex is not just to service men's sexual wishes and that sex should be a pleasurable and safe activity for women too

I think all women (with and without learning disabilities) need *all* these things. It is clear to those who work closely with women with learning disabilities that some don't have *any* of these things. I have only met one who has. As far as I can see, HIV prevention work with women with learning disabilities needs to address all the above issues and will fail if it concentrates solely on the provision of information about HIV and condoms.

Working with Men with Learning Disabilities

I wrote in the introduction that men with learning disabilities have the power to practice safer sex, but usually not the motivation. That they have power is apparent from what has been said here and elsewhere about the control they almost always have when they have sex with women with learning disabilities. There is also the obvious point that condoms go on penises and if they wanted to put one on, there would be no one to stop them. It is therefore necessary to look in more detail at motivation. Men with and without learning disabilities have traditionally not taken responsibility for precautions to do with sex. Contraception has largely been the woman's responsibility. For the vast majority of men with learning disabilities, including all the men the Sex Education Team has worked with, little or no interest or responsibility has been taken for contraception.

In our work we have met no men with learning disabilities who have sex exclusively with women who have ever had a sexually transmitted disease. This compares to a small number of women with learning disabilities who have had a sexually transmitted disease and who know that it came from having sex with a man. The experience of the vast majority of men with learning disabilities is therefore likely not to include any physiological consequences of sex with women. It is usually very difficult to try to persuade them otherwise. It is difficult to shift the men from their position that nothing is going to happen or that this is not a serious issue for them, a difficult position to challenge because you can not imply that they will or are likely to get HIV. Their lack of motivation is not entirely unreasonable, given that the chances of HIV infection from a woman with learning disabilities are very slim indeed. The decision to be honest about the small risk or to overemphasise it (Young Adult Institute, 1987) is one that all safer sex advisors have to take.

Another issue to be taken into account is that men with learning disabilities, who are almost always the ones to take the initiative sexually, have known for many years that staff, parents or other people in society actually do not want them to have sex. The message has usually been crystal clear in the past, yet many men with learning disabilities ignore that message. I am not implying that they remain unaffected by it on a psychological or emotional level, but that they actively seek and have sex regardless of the message. Whatever our role therefore, we cannot expect that they will necessarily take any notice of this new message. Safer sex messages do not come from or go into a vacuum, rather a context where past sexual messages have been negative, stigmatising and punishing. It is very important to understand this process and not to make harsh judgements about people who seem not to want to take our good advice.

As with women, it is just as important to find out what kinds of sex the man is having and with whom. What this will probably reveal is that he is definitely having vaginal and probably also anal penetrative sex. Given that almost all women with learning disabilities we have met have said they do not like anal sex and because it is potentially painful, we have encouraged men who have sex with women not to do it. This is a good example of not just being concerned about reducing HIV risk and we have also tried to act as advocates for individual women with learning disabilities directly through our work with them and indirectly in our work with men.

My male colleagues have felt it a priority to work with the issue of HIV and safer sex in a very much broader context with men with learning disabilities. Men cannot be encouraged to think of their own and their partner's sexual

93

health without thinking about their own and their partner's feelings and reasons for having sex. Men with learning disabilities very often do not know whether the woman likes sex with them or, if she does, what kinds of sex she likes and dislikes (McCarthy & Thompson, 1993). Consequently they will be encouraged to actually ask the woman. Although this might seem very artificial behaviour we know of men and women with learning disabilities who have been having sex together for many years and still don't give out or pick up signals about what is and isn't OK. The advice is not always accepted or put into action, but he will at least have been given a clear message that it is unacceptable to have sex without considering his partners' feelings. Many men with learning disabilities who have sex with women also have sex with men. This raises issues about sexual identity and whether it is appropriate to explore that aspect. On the whole that has not been tackled, owing to its complexity and doubts about it's worth (Thompson, 1994). However, the men are prompted to consider what the women (who are publicly and privately acknowledged as having the special status of girlfriend) might think about it. The men usually know that the women would not like it if they knew.

Concluding Remarks

I would have ideally liked to have finished this chapter by giving examples of safer sex teaching which was successful in the sense that people with learning disabilities were regularly having safer sex as a result of the educational inputs. Unfortunately I have to say that we do not have much confidence that this has been the outcome for any more than a small minority of the people we have worked with. In this complex area of work, however, it is important to take a broad view of what constitutes success. For example, is it a mark of success to have given people with learning disabilities an opportunity to talk about their sexual experiences in an adult and respectful way, possibly for the first time in their lives? The answer has to be yes.

Success is also educating people that they have rights and responsibilities and that other people should not treat them badly. Letting people know they are valued and trying to raise people's self esteem in order that they might be able to learn how to take care of themselves is also a positive intervention. Most importantly, success is letting people with learning disabilities know that the difficulties they face with sex and safer sex are problems shared by many other people and are not simply their shortcomings as individuals.

It is unrealistic to expect all or even most people with learning disabilities to be able or willing to always practice safer sex as a result of having been educated about risk. This is after all, not the case for the general population, nor particular groups of the population at increased risk (Fitzpatrick et al., 1989). However, if we establish trust and facilitate communication with people with learning disabilities, then hope exists to enable them to make more informed choices about their sexual lives and the risk of HIV. Even in the short term, at least people will have received information and support regarding sex and safer sex which they would not otherwise have had. Without information and support there is little hope of people making good decisions and important changes. With information, support and encouragement, the potential for change exists.

References

Finch, J. (1984) *It's great to have someone to talk to: the ethics and politics of interviewing women.* In C. Bell, & H. Roberts, (eds.) Social researching: politics, problems and practice. London: Routledge & Kegan Paul.

Fitzpatrick, R., Bolton, M. & Hart, C. (1989) *Gay men's sexual behaviour in response to AIDS: insights and problems.* In A. Aggleton, et al. (eds.) AIDS: social representations, social practices. Lewes: Falmer Press.

Jacobs, R., Samovitz,P., Levy, J & Levy, P. (1989) *Developing an AIDS Prevention education programme for persons with developmental disabilities.* Mental Retardation, 24,4; 233-7.

McCarthy, M. (1993) *Sexual experiences of women with learning difficulties in longstay hospitals.* Sexuality and Disability, 11, 4: 277-285.

McCarthy, M. (1994) *Against All Odds: HIV and safer sex education with women with learning difficulties.* In L. Doyal, et al. (eds.) AIDS: Setting a feminist agenda. London : Taylor and Francis.

McCarthy, M. & Thompson, D. (1993) *Sex and the 3 R's rights, responsibilities and risks.* Brighton Pavilion.

McCarthy, M. & Thompson, D. (1994) *HIV/AIDS and safer sex work with people with learning disabilities.* In A. Craft, (ed.) Practice Issues in Sexuality and Learning Disabilities. London : Routledge.

Oakley, A. (1981)   *Interviewing women: a contradiction in terms.* In H. Roberts, (ed.) Doing Feminist Research. London: Routledge and Kegan Paul.

O'Sullivan, A. &   *You, Me and HIV.* Cambridge: Daniels Publishing.
Gillies,P. (1993)

People First   *Everything you ever wanted to know about safer sex....*
(undated)   London: People First.

Rees, S. &   *An educational programme on HIV for formerly institutionalised*
Berchert, R. (1992) *people with developmental disabilities.* In A. Crocker, et al. (eds.) HIV infection and developmental disabilities: a resource for service providers. Baltimore: Paul H. Brookes Publishing.

Thompson, D.   *Personal Communication.*
(1994)

Thompson, D.   *Sexual experience and sexual identity for men with learning disabilities*
(1994)   *who have sex with men.* Changes: an international journal of psychology and psychotherapy, 12, 4: 254-263

Young Adult   *Teaching People with Disabilities to Better Protect Themselves*
Institute (1987)   New York.

Michelle McCarthy is Lecturer in Learning Disability and Service Development Consultant at the Tizard Centre, University of Kent at Canterbury. For four years she was Team Leader of the Sex Education Team at Harperbury, providing a specialist sexuality service to people with learning disabilities and staff. Michelle's particular interests are working with women with learning disabilities on issues of sexual abuse and sexual health.

Chapter 7

Experiences of Risk - The Role of Therapy in Sexual Health

by Stephen Morris

Introduction

There is a range of approaches to counselling and therapy which place different emphasis on thoughts, feelings and behaviours. Psychodynamic theories and approaches work with feelings and beliefs to:

'explore the boundary between what happens in the real world and how this is perceived and encoded in the internal fantasy and emotional life of the individual' (Smith & Brown, 1992, p. 86)

Some practitioners choose to address issues of risk-taking only at the more concrete levels of choices, knowledge and changing behaviour. In our work at Respond, we have come to see powerful and sometimes chaotic patterns beyond the low self esteem and distorted beliefs about sexuality which such approaches target. This account may appear dramatic to people who are unused to psychotherapeutic discourse, but it invites you to suspend the disbelief you may have in order to allow an appreciation of the extreme feelings which are aroused by both real and feared trauma in the lives and experiences of people with learning disabilities.

Dangerousness, Risk and Sexual Health

Danger and dangerousness are central features of the human condition, so much so in fact, that it is easy to conclude that the very act of living is dangerous. From conception the threat to life exists in many forms. Protection against danger requires both physical and psychic resources and much of our conscious and unconscious life is engaged in protecting and defending against real and imagined dangers. The threat to health and to life represented by HIV and AIDS encapsulates many aspects of danger and dangerousness for large groups of the population and the association of dangerous behaviour with sex, which is also fundamental to the human condition, creates a terrifying challenge to our psychic and physical resources. This conscious and unconscious trauma is reinforced by health promotion messages which convey considerations of risk and responsibility and social and media messages which both reinforce and compromise these.

Our creative responses to this aspect of the human condition are usually highly effective, with practical measures and psychic interventions such as defence and denial, enabling us to maintain a sense of safety, well being and healthy equilibrium. Maintenance of this equilibrium is however fraught with risk and when the reality of danger and dangerousness manifest in whatever form, the consequences can have a major impact on mental health. People with learning disabilities are particularly likely to experience a powerful threat to their sense of safety and healthy equilibrium. It is difficult to think of any other group in our society which is confronted so painfully at all stages of its development with the ultimate danger of annihilation.

The threat of annihilation experienced by people with learning disabilities has particular significance for the responses of people working with them, especially in the field of sexual health counselling and psychotherapy. Recognition of the importance of the sexual health of people with learning disabilities is now widespread and many initiatives have been developed in response. The pioneering and inspiring work of Ann Craft (1987) had a dramatic impact. Craft opened our eyes to the fact that people with learning disabilities were also sexual beings and in so doing, enabled some of the most taboo and therefore potentially dangerous issues to be faced. Sexual health work with people with learning disabilities continues to confront these issues and as this chapter will make clear, key aspects of sexual health work involve considering other challenging areas of the human condition, including considerations of life and death. It is only when we can bear to recognise that all sexual health work touches on these issues that we can begin to appreciate fully the real nature of danger, dangerousness and the consequential risks involved in sexual activity.

The reality of the risk of annihilation as experienced by people with learning disabilities has featured in all my work. In the early 1980s, I began to consult on sex education to staff groups of day care and residential workers. These events were often planned to include the whole staff team, although it was not unusual for only a small number of the staff group to attend. Those who did would confront me repeatedly with the same question, namely 'isn't this work dangerous?' or by implication, stating 'We cannot do sex education work, it's too dangerous'. Throughout the country the response was the same. When asking the groups to define the danger they would usually begin by talking about risk, but no one would be able to define the precise nature of this risk or the perceived danger. It was later in my direct clinical work with people with learning disabilities that the real meaning and source of these feelings was found.

Developing a Psychoanalytic Approach

Following a series of sex education workshops in which I worked with small groups of people with learning disabilities, I decided to take a representative sample of those attending and to test their ability to integrate and to use the knowledge provided to them. The results were disappointing, as little information had been remembered and some were still engaging in dangerous sexual activity. As a consequence, I decided to move from a cognitive to a more analytic approach to intervention. Rather than following a set agenda, I decided to work with whatever issues individuals brought to the group. Where possible these issues would be related to feelings, self esteem and personal history and then to concrete information giving about sex, sexuality and relationships. The results were very different. Participants engaged fully in the process, attendance was constant and concrete changes in life style were evident. However, there were other factors in this process that gave meaning to the feelings of danger and risk identified by so many anxious staff groups. This was to have far reaching consequences for the future provision of sex education and work addressing issues of sexual health.

In psychoanalytic practice, recognition and respect of feeling, experience and life history enable clients to communicate both the conscious and unconscious material of their lives. My new approach to the sex education groups facilitated communication and in so doing, revealed horrific and painful experiences of trauma. Many people attending the groups, when feeling safe enough to communicate, told of experiences of emotional, physical and sexual abuse. However, all those attending the groups communicated without exception, the trauma of being born with a learning disability. As one young man put it and similar to how many others have described their birth experience 'I came out wrong'. The impact of the belief that you 'came out wrong', confirmed by organic features of learning disability, results in a defined experience of trauma for both the baby and its carers. It is the experience of trauma, having been suppressed sometimes for many years, that confronts the sexual health worker. Often without realising it, they will begin to talk about sex, the very

99

cause of the trauma itself.

In clinical practice with people with learning disabilities, talking about sex ultimately develops into talking about disability, birth, death (Morris, 1994) It is essential that we understand why this is so. Such an understanding will not only assist in overcoming the fears that so often prevent sex education from being provided but, perhaps more importantly, help us to recognise and address some of the dangerous sexual behaviour exhibited by many of our clients and to begin to treat post traumatic stress disorders.

Learned Pathology

During several episodes of a well known television soap opera, two characters openly discussed the dilemma of having a baby with Down's Syndrome. The option of having the handicapped baby aborted was portrayed as a favourable and positive choice. Several of my clients in their weekly psychotherapy session talked about this and revealed how aware they were about the wish of many in society to eradicate difference when it manifests in the form of handicap. I was reminded of the many occasions during sex education sessions when watching the birth of a baby on video, how the participants would follow the discussion with their stories of loss and bereavement. Experiencing the death wish of the world around them, be it expressed as openly as in the television soap or in less explicit ways, is a constant reminder to people with learning disabilities that something terrible happened at birth (Morris, 1995; Rock, 1996). If something terrible came out wrong then something terrible must have been done to create it. The latter belief is again echoed by many of my clients in both individual and group psychotherapy.

Piontelli, in her book *From Foetus to Child* (1992), provides several accounts of her observations of foetus in utero. These psychoanalytic foetal observations provide a moving account of how external environmental events have an effect on the foetus and illustrates how behaviours in the womb can still be observed in the child's developing years. Environmental influences undoubtedly impact directly on the unborn child and on its maternal attachment. When that process includes feelings and emotions of fear, hate, murderous rage and rejection, the threat of annihilation becomes, if not an external reality, a psychic reality. One of the first risks the sexual health worker must face and prepare for in working with people with learning disabilities is the risk that in opening up the issue of sex and sexuality, powerful and

100

painful trauma about the client's very existence will also surface. The connection between sex and death is central.

Enabling a client to communicate fears, fantasies and thoughts about their conception, birth and life will facilitate a mourning process and eventually enable the integration of a healthy self-esteem and sense of self. Without this process sexual health for the learning disabled client may not be possible as the perceived threat of annihilation will be constantly experienced in connection with sexual functioning.

More than Sex Education

The dangers and risks presented in supervision and consultancies by carers often reflect the consequences of this with the further consequence that responses focus on issues of control, choice and freedom. Although these are important issues, the behaviours we find ourselves trying to address are often symptomatic of the double trauma this chapter has so far focused on. Compulsive sexual activity, sexual disregard of others, sexualised self-harm and sexual harm of others are all symptoms that require more than sex *education*. Indeed, it may not be possible to address these areas of danger and risk at all by the provision of sex education alone. These behaviours are manifesting not because the person does not *know* any different or solely because they are learning disabled. Rather, the behaviours are *enactments of what cannot be said*: sex holds the risk of annihilation.

Many of the behaviours that come to the attention of the sexual health worker result in referral to psychotherapy and include behaviours that involve varying degrees of risk and dangerousness. Sometimes these behaviours can be defined as criminal and many of the behaviours involve the harming of self or others. Freud (1901), asserted that thoughts and fantasies are symbolic representations of actions and that actions are symbolic representations of thoughts. As James Gilligan (1996) points out, when writing about shame in special settings, actions can proceed and serve as substitutes for words. At Respond, we see many men and women whose lives have been impaired with the perceived threat of annihilation and the social consequences of learning disability, the main features of which are often loneliness and isolation. It is not just past unspeakable traumas that contribute to disturbed acting out behaviours but also the social impoverishment of having no one to communicate with. What is the point of words when what you have to say is too painful and worse still, when there is no one to hear you. Acting out what cannot be said involves some of the most dangerous and risky behaviours possible, as they often put life itself at risk. The following behaviours are taken from a small sample of referrals for psychotherapy: compulsive masturbation using auto-phixia techniques; inserting sharp objects into the vagina; having unprotected sex in public toilets; raping a women at knife point; refusing to wear condoms when engaging in anal sex; paedophilic sex using threat of murder; sexual assault on homeless males; forcing young women at a day centre to have unprotected sex in the toilet; and, forcing a current partner to have unprotected sex. These sexual behaviours also involve the threat or actual acts of aggression and violence. What also becomes obvious in the course of treatment is that these acts also involve for the perpetrator, powerful elements of pleasure. It is the experience of pleasure that makes highly dangerous behaviour addictive and compulsive and further indicates the reason for the need to repeatedly act them out.

Recognising Perversion

My clinical work with people who present with disturbed sexual health which also carries sexual health implications has confirmed for me the presence of perversion. Recognising the specific diagnostic features of perversion, free from the moral connotations of the word, enable dangerousness and risk to be addressed directly through treatment. Making a careful assessment on referral is important for determining what is required in terms of treatment and education. Many of those referred because of concerns about their sexual health do not require therapy. A clear and comprehensive sex education that recognises the importance of feelings, emotions and self esteem can have an immediate impact, with many positive outcomes. However, because the incidence of sexual trauma is high in this group and because trauma is associated with the threat and fantasy of annihilation, the development of perversion is perhaps more common than we would like to believe.

Estela Welldon of the Portman Clinic, London (1996), explains that perversion involves a deep split between genital mature sexuality as a living or loving force, and what appears to be sexual, but what in fact corresponds to much more primitive stages of development which are pervasively dominated by pregenitality. Achievement of intimacy with another partner through sexual intercourse is replaced in perversion by release from increasing sexual anxiety through bizarre action or situations which in themselves are inexplicable not only to others but also to the person involved. Robert Stoller (1975) draws attention to the element of hostility within perversion and explains that the presence of hostility takes form in a fantasy of revenge hidden in the actions that make up the perversion, serving to convert childhood trauma into adult triumph. He also points out that to create the greatest excitement, the perversion must also portray itself as an act of risk taking.

The level of sexual anxiety in many people with learning disabilities is high and related directly to the primitive experiences of their conception that they connect with through fantasy, and as illustrated earlier, by concrete experience of the external world. When cognitive deficits makes the working through of such trauma difficult, the service of one's own sexual and libidinal energy to reduce anxiety and enable past experiences of powerlessness to be experienced from a position of triumph, becomes a useful resource and a powerful defence. When diagnosing perversion, Welldon (1996) explains that the following psycho-dynamic and phenomenological features of a client's personality structure should be present

1. that the perverse action involves repetition and compulsion and provides release of sexual anxiety

2. although the client is aware of the need to repeat the act there is no awareness of its hostile component - it is only in treatment that the presence of hate and revenge become clear

3. a true sexual perversion involves the body and does not stay in the realm of fantasy: the sexual action usually is fixed and repetitive

4. the other person is experienced as a 'part object' rather than as a whole and separate person; other features involve an inability to see themselves as a separate being, and

5. there is often an extreme fear of being trapped and an overwhelming need to be in complete control; actions often involve hostility and humiliation directed at others or themselves.

Within the sex offender group therapy programme at Respond these characteristics are much in evidence. The process of making a traumatic experience a triumphant one permeates all aspects of the lives of those attending, and can be seen to be employed on a daily basis. For example, when the time to start the group was changed because of external reasons the group members made the imposed decision their own by fantasising that they had made the decision the week before.

Therapeutic Response and Intervention

The opportunity exists in individual treatment for the dangerous behaviour to become recognised and considered in relation to other aspects of the client's life. Until this happens it is usually separated off and secret, giving rise to guilt, fear and increased anxiety which act as a motor and maintain a circular process. Individual psychotherapy can provide the experience of a safe and non-perverse relationship. There are many risks the client has to face in commencing treatment when past experiences of closeness and intimacy have resulted in traumatic experiences of abuse, deprivation and humiliation. The intimacy of the therapeutic relationship can increase the anxiety of annihilation. Support and sometimes safe containment outside the therapy is essential.

When on-going treatment in psychotherapy is required it should not be provided in isolation. A multi-disciplinary and multi-agency approach is essential in the understanding, recognition and reduction of the risks and dangers such clients present. Good communication and networking between agencies is also essential if treatment or education are to be fully effective. One of the first tasks facing the sex educator, counsellor or psychotherapist is to make an assessment of the existing network and of the client's history. Welldon (1996) refers to Stoller (1991) when highlighting that when working with trauma and trauma related perversions, it is important to recognise fully and work with influences across a three generational process. Stoller, (1991) has observed that battered children grow up to be battering parents, that paedophiles were sexually molested boys and that serial rapists were often victims of forced or exploitative erotic abuse in boyhood. Although such links are by no means inevitable (Brown & Thompson, in press), tracing the origins of trauma in clients attending Respond for treatment often reveal an alarming degree of intergenerational abuse and deprivation and commencing therapy is often the only opportunity which offers the possibility of breaking the vicious cycle.

When clients draw attention to trauma by acting out what has been done to them there is a very real risk that professionals will not recognise the true nature of the unconscious communication. Reluctance to name presenting symptoms, for what they are, is common and is one of the most dangerous responses. It is not unusual when consulting to hear professionals describe their client who is violently raping or explicitly sexually assaulting others as 'engaging in sexually inappropriate behaviour'. Often many attempts have been made to educate the client sexually, but naming what the client is communicating is the first step in reducing risk, including the risk of HIV infection and letting the client know that what they are communicating is being recognised. Minimising the reality of what the client is doing also minimises the opportunity for treatment.

Recognition of minute detail is also important. Stoller, in *Perversion - the Erotic Form of Hatred* (1975), illustrates this by citing how the content of pornographic material used by one of his patients reflected not only key features of the client's perverse behaviour but also symbolised aspects of the past trauma (see also Millar, 1987). The process of intensive risk assessment will enable detailed information to be revealed and considered in this way. Risk assessment prior to education or treatment is therefore recommended. A thorough risk assessment should identify not only what level of risk and danger the client presents to others but also explicitly *what* is risky and dangerous for the client. One paedophile in treatment with me was given opportunities to offend because his day care programme came to an end each day at 3.30pm. He travelled home on public transport and used a bus route that passed several schools. This particular man was very resistant to treatment but recognition of how external factors contributed to his offending helped reduce the risk he and his time-table posed. This example also illustrates how total confidentiality when working with such issues is not possible. Conditions of limited confidentiality are required for the safety of all concerned.

Responding to HIV Risk

In order to help to ensure safety and reduce risk, practical intervention is also usually required. Interventions in the realm of sexual health and sexual well-being are particularly challenging to all professionals working with adults with learning disabilities. Not only is a clear legal framework absent, but the very issues concerning the intervention are themselves symptomatic of the learning disabled person's experience of powerlessness. When professionals get caught up in the process of treatment, case-work, care planning and other task centred interventions, it becomes progressively easier to forget or fail to recognise the pain and suffering of the person concerned.

Clients who are led to act out their distress and past trauma sexually are deeply unhappy people who are fighting for their survival. This needs to be emphasised, as it is seldom recognised to be the case. When faced with the unbearable, it is not uncommon for people in caring or support roles to get caught up in the desire to punish and control, as there may also be an unconscious desire to remove that which causes distress. As a clinician, with responsibility for taking referrals for treatment, it is easy to recognise the hostility with which some referrals are made. During assessment it is possible to detect both the conscious and unconscious processes present in a client's support network. In recognising these, it is often necessary for the first intervention to be directed at the professional network rather than the client. Therapeutic intervention will be ineffective if the other people involved with the person are full of anger or unconscious murderous intent.

Dangerous, controlling and occasionally sadistic 'professional' interventions can be identified in many areas of this work and these tend to bear the unconscious hallmark of annihilation. When the issue of HIV or AIDS is present such hallmarks are even more visible. People with learning disabilities who are sexually active and have not received education, support and access to protective resources are clearly at risk. They are also at risk and sometimes at the mercy of a neo-fascist morality which is occasionally viciously implemented by some of those who enact powerful roles or who occupy 'professional' positions. I will take the case of a young man for whom we will use the pseudonym Adam, who was brought to see me against his will, to illustrate this observation. He was known to be sexually active with both men and women. He accessed the wider community with skill, occasionally visited prostitutes and regularly used pornography as a stimulus for private masturbation.

Very early in his assessment it was clear that his sexual functioning was serving as a defence against past trauma. His sexual activity was compulsive and involved sado-masochistic fantasies which were frequently acted out, with his sexual objects tied up before intercourse. As typical in true perversion, these elements of his sexual acting out were secret and until he commenced treatment were known only by him. He was therefore not referred because of the nature of his sexual activity but because of the expressed concern and belief of those supporting him that he was putting others at risk of HIV infection. The reality was however, very different. Adam was scrupulous in his practice of safer sex. He always used a condom and insisted that the people he had sex with used one as well. His real risks were at the core of his perversion and did not involve the risk of HIV infection. The real risk for him was not having access to his sexual acting out. Consciously, he did all he could to remain healthy, as he understood this was important if he was able to maintain his defence against past trauma, namely trauma turned to triumph by being acted out through sado-masochism.

Adam came into treatment just in time. I discovered that because of the professional perception of risk, a twenty-four hour regime of control had been established around him. He was never alone and was not allowed to use pornography, even in private. As a consequence, all his sexual activity was curtailed. His defences had been unwittingly removed and he was very close to suffering deep clinical depression. Without resources to work through his past traumas and without his defences, this young man would have suffered serious mental ill health or committed suicide. In discussions with his support network, it was evident that those involved in his care held extremely negative feelings towards him, so much so that the extent that his pain and the real risks involved were not allowed to be communicated. Adam has now been in treatment for three years and the source of his pain has been acknowledged without him having to resort to acting out. Those supporting him now recognise the real nature of risk and are enabling him to enjoy healthy sexual fulfilment, free from inappropriate restrictions.

Another man for whom I will use the pseudonym Peter, does present a real sexual health risk to himself and others. Peter has anal sex with men, usually strangers, in a number of public toilets, car parks, parks and public gardens. He refuses to use condoms and doesn't mind if others having sex with him don't use them either. Peter's behaviour is not uncommon and whilst the process of psychotherapy can address his unconscious destructive wishes and help him understand why he behaves in such a way, it cannot at once make him safe. When faced with such worrying and high risk behaviour, some professionals have sought to implement total control over an individual's life. Whilst responding to one moral dilemma, such action also presents new dilemmas, highlighting once again the powerlessness people with learning disabilities are vulnerable to. Others in society who are not learning disabled may engage in unsafe sexual behaviours and at present, are rarely prevented from doing so.

Psychotherapy can achieve an internal change that would enable someone like Peter, to value his own life and the lives of others. Psychotherapeutic interventions are not a magic cure, but over a period of time, can facilitate change and healing. When clients like Adam and Peter present their needs, pain and particular individual challenges, a variety of interventions are required. Any intervention working in isolation is potentially dangerous, but psychotherapists working with sex educators, health workers and teachers can help provide an effective combination.

Conclusion

People with learning disabilities are constantly at risk of being characterised and determined by massive exposure to anxiety, threat of annihilation, abuse, trauma and deprivation, all of which have the potential of being acted out in risk taking, self negating or abusing behaviours. This is as evident for dangerousness and the risk of HIV infection to self and others as it is to dangerousness and risk in relation to abusive sexual behaviours. The resource of counselling and psychotherapy, when combined with sexual health and educational interventions can offer understanding and interpretation of this link. Psychotherapy as a treatment is essential when risk and danger have become a reality.

References

Brown, H. &   *A minefield in a vacuum: the ethics of working with men with*
Thompson, D.   *learning disabilities who have unacceptable or abusive sexual*
(in press)   *behaviours*, Disability and Society.

Craft, A. (1987) 'Mental handicap and sexuality: issues for individuals with a
                  mental handicap, their parents and professionals', in A. Craft,
                  (ed.) Mental Handicap and Sexuality: Issues and
                  Perspectives, Costello, Tunbridge Wells.

Freud, S. (1901) 'The psychopathology of everyday life' In J. Strachey (ed.) The
                  Standard Edition of the Complete Psychological Works of
                  Sigmund Freud, Vol 6, Hogarth Press, London.

Cilligan, J. (1996) 'Exploring shame in special settings' In C. Cordess and M.Cox
                  (ed.) Forensic Psychotherapy - Crime Psychodynamics and the
                  Offender Patient - Vol 2 Jessica Kingsley, London.

Millar, A (1987) *For your own good: the roots of violence in child rearing*, Virago
                  Press, London.

Morris, S. (1994) 'From Denial to Justice' - Paper presented to the Nexus annual
                  conference - Belfast.

Morris, S. (1995) 'Clinical Examples of Primal Scene Experience' - Paper presented
                  to the Freud Seminar - Centre for Attachment Based
                  Psychoanalytic Psychotherapy London.

Piontelli, A.(1992) 'From Foetus to Child An observational and psychoanalytic
                  study', Routledge, London.

Rock, P.(1996)   *Eugenics and Euthanasia: a case for concern for disabled people,
                  particularly disabled women.* Disability and Society, Vol.11,
                  March, pp. 121-129.

Smith, H. &   *Inside out: a psychodynamic approach to normalisation*, in (Eds.)
Brown, H. (1992) H. Brown and H. Smith, Normalisation: a Reader for the
                  Nineties, Routledge, London.

Stoller, R. (1975) 'Perversion - the erotic form of hatred', Karnac Books, London.

Stoller, R. (1991)   '*The term perversion*', in, (Eds.) C. Fogel and W. Myers, Perversions and Near Perversions. New Haven, CT; Yale University Press.

Welldon, E. (1996)   '*Contrasts in male and female sexual perversions*' in (Eds.) C. Cordess and M. Cox, Forensic Psychotherapy, Jessica Kingsley, London.

Stephen Morris is co-founder and Clinical Director of Respond, an agency providing individual and group psychotherapy to people with learning disabilities who have been sexually abused and who sexually abuse. It is the only forensic service in the United Kingdom working solely with people with learning disabilities. Respond offers a range of clinical services including treatment programmes, risk assessment, investigative interviewing, training, consultancy and supervision.

Chapter 8

Safer Sex Training for Peer Educators

by Fiona Barber and Paul Redfern

Introduction

'All teaching in all subjects aims to stimulate interest. It would be odd if this were not true of sex lessons' (Probert, 1973, quoted in Metcalfe 1989, p. 231).

In 1994, the Wandsworth Area Health Authority agreed to fund a project to enable people with learning disabilities to train others about safer sex. The idea was that a group of people with learning disabilities would then work alongside some professionals and visit residential or day support services to present ideas about safer sex to other people with learning disabilities. Respond (see Chapter 7 by Stephen Morris) were given the tender for the Safer Sex for Peers Training Course.

Respond had already been working with several of the peer educators about aspects of sex and had encountered much evidence of sexual abuse by other people with learning disabilities and by people entrusted with the care and support of people with learning disabilities. Counselling was on offer as part of this service and Respond aimed to empower people with learning disabilities to make choices about what services they received and how to use them.

Fiona Barber, a qualified social worker in Croydon, was already working at Respond when Stephen Morris approached her about taking on the responsibility of piloting the course. She in turn approached Paul Redfern, an established trainer in the field of deafness, who had already been part of a project team in the writing of a Training the Trainers course for the Local Government Training Board, to co-tutor the course.

It was subsequently agreed that Respond would host a one week peer education training course for people who had already attended courses about safer sex. It was hoped that the applicants would have a sound knowledge of what sex is about and how to engage in safer sex. The weeks training would offer revision and update on HIV and AIDS in response to any needs identified and include training on presentation skills. The week would then be followed up with a workshop where professionals (who had been on similar courses elsewhere) and participants would meet and make connections and plans for working together.

Philosophies and Approaches

We both held complementary views about how best to approach the task.

Fiona Barber: Involving people with learning disabilities in the education and training of their peers seemed a most effective way of empowering people. I was aware that they are devalued and infantilised by the services and support systems created to meet their needs. This is reinforced and compounded by the families and communities in which they live. The notion of the right to a sexual self has a mixed reception throughout those families, communities and systems. I do not believe that ignorance is bliss and feel that disadvantaged groups are the last ones to gain access to the information they need to obtain their rights. I was therefore immediately interested in being a part of this project.

Paul Redfern: As a deaf person, I was initially nervous about taking this kind of work on, having only previously experienced working with people with learning disabilities who were deaf. I envisaged a number of communication problems although I am able to lipread well and have mostly recognisable speech, as well as having British Sign Language as a second language. As a consequence of these considerations, I was initially unsure as to whether I was an appropriate person to do the work. However, the key quality that had attracted Steve and Fiona was that I had done a lot of work around teaching people in presentation and training skills, that I was an established writer and communicator and had knowledge of HIV and AIDS and safer sex.

My view was and remains fundamentally straightforward. People with learning disabilities have the right to make the same choices as anyone else in our community as to how they live, work and play. The project appealed to me, because having worked as a social services training officer for a London borough, I knew how many people were 'cared for'. On closer examination, this care often proves to be a form of containment where few choices are made available. My view is that a lack of choices in lifestyle inevitably leads to a narrow range of options for sexual activity. Denial of information and choices, to my mind, does not de-sexualise people with learning disabilities, rather it puts them at greater risk.

Preparation

We both invested much time discussing our respective philosophies in order that we could develop and present a consistent and united front during the training week. It was hoped that this would prevent contradictory messages being sent out either directly or indirectly. We also needed to feel safe about working together and resolve any personal anxieties in order that we did not project our own fears onto participants. Despite being bombarded with sexual messages by the media, many of which are frankly titillating and overtly sexist (and by omission, homophobic), it still proves difficult to discuss sex rationally in our society and any discussion is often unwelcome. After much debate we agreed to start from the premise that sex is a risky venture, not just in physical or health terms but also emotionally. People are right to talk about safer sex rather than safe sex, because no sexual contact is entirely safe in terms of physical (and certainly emotional) health. However, we also felt strongly that people engage in sexual activity for a variety of reasons, and personal enjoyment is a strong motivating factor.

To avoid a 'doom and gloom' approach (we definitely did not want to send out overly negative messages about sex) we aimed to work from this premise and convey sex in terms of enjoyment as well as risk. We decided to look at safety under three categories.

* safety from unwanted sex

* safety from unwanted pregnancy

* safety from HIV infection or other STDs

We wanted to provide a major focus on self advocacy. The research shows that many people with learning disabilities have been recipients of sexual abuse or exploitation (Brown, Stein & Turk, 1995). We therefore wanted the course to have a strong emphasis on participants being able to join in or opt out freely and to make choices, both out of principle but also because many will have experienced unwanted sex. Participants should have the right to say Yes or No in every aspect of their lives. We accordingly designed the course as a model of decision-making to encourage people to advocate for themselves and possibly others later on.

We were prepared to encounter some nervousness about the subject. Some participants might be overly anxious about offending us or reticent to

113

use words that they had been told were bad or should not be used. Our view was that if a word was more easily understood, then they should choose what they wanted to use rather than the professionally or technically correct one.

When discussing the administration of the course with Respond, it was agreed that all participants would be self-selecting, with application forms filled out and sent in. There would be no interview procedure. The major reason was to avoid any form of selection which might be based on an unconscious idea of what constituted the right sort of participant. It was also agreed that the course would be oriented towards training rather than groupwork. Many of the participants had already attended groups in the past and experience suggested that maintaining boundaries might be difficult if this distinction was not made. If participants were to train their peers about safer sex, we felt that the concept of training needed to be clearly defined and the question of boundaries would have to be addressed early in the process. The aim was simple: the course would equip them with the skills needed to work as co-trainers.

It remained important however, not to take anything for granted, and we needed to check out how much they actually did remember from other courses or their groups. We also agreed to make the course as interactive as possible, developing portfolios which each person could build on and take home if they wished. This area of work was heavily dependent on pictures and their own written contributions, the aim being to offer a reference source for any future development work they undertook.

Because Paul is deaf and because of the nature of the course and subject, we determined that the course would need communication rules as well as ground rules. Box 1 lists the set of communication rules and Box 2 the set of ground rules developed to guide the work.

BOX I
COMMUNICATION RULES

- One person to communicate at a time

- Show your hand when you want to talk

- Ask if you don't understand

- Look at people when you talk to them

- Use some signs to help each other

- Maintain eye contact

- Don't say it's okay when it's not

- Speak clearly and remember Paul needs to see your face

BOX 2
GROUND RULES

- Don't talk outside about people's personal problems

- Do talk about safer sex

- Be here on time

- Be neat and tidy

- It's okay to be embarrassed

- Don't make fun of others

- Don't ask personal questions

- Don't talk behind each other's backs

- You don't have to answer personal questions

Organisation

One question was how to organise the thirty hours which had been allocated for the course. The decision was made to opt for a five day week block course. We found this format helpful for a number of reasons.

A block course emphasised the difference between groupwork (which was based on the weekly two-hourly model) and training and helped keep up the momentum for open discussion. All the participants had already been involved with groups and we were able to discuss the difference between training and being in a group. Some issues were of course the same, such as confidentiality and respect, but it was felt important for participants to know that our course was primarily an opportunity for learning and to transfer the knowledge learnt.

We agreed to keep a diary of each day (apart from Friday, when we were too tired to make notes!) so that we could alter session plans according to what we felt was required by the participants. It also gave us the information we needed to help us review the week as it progressed (names have been changed in relation to the excerpts in the diaries).

The Course

We learnt very quickly that many participants were vague about some of the rudiments of sex despite having been on other courses. In particular some displayed a very low level of understanding of how their bodies worked (Box 3). We soon realised the original aim of training people to become co-trainers was unlikely to be realised within the time-scales set. The original plan included some training techniques, such as presentation skills. These were now felt inappropriate for the level of comprehension reached about safer sex, therefore it was decided to concentrate on empowering participants to make a decision on whether they wanted to continue with this kind of training.

Participants may have been vague about several aspects about sex or safer sex but they were clear about HIV and AIDS. Like many people, these two concepts filled them with dread and horror. What HIV actually is and how it is contracted had not been explained in terms that could be retained. One person grasped the concept that a syringe could transmit HIV but could not differentiate between the contexts in which the syringe was used.

There was clearly a gender difference in understanding contraception. The women were clear about how to use the different varieties and the purpose of contraception while the man was completely unaware of what contraception was. If this is replicated (and there is evidence from sex education groupwork that this tends to be the case), it suggests a substantive difference in emphasis on contraception and this left us feeling uneasy at the implications. One possible implication is that women with learning disabilities are controlled by parents, staff and others who do not want them to conceive. There is therefore a strong emphasis on preventing conception but a lack of information on how to have a fulfilling sex life. This concern was reinforced by the fact that none of the participants appeared to be experienced in handling condoms or femidoms. An excerpt from the diary notes shows this clearly:

'Some people had problems trying to read the date mark on the condom packets, and in finding the Kitemark, but they all chose a packet to open and practice on a courgette very happily. They tried twice, Ms F was flustered and angry at being shown how to do it, she insisted she didn't need help, but in fact she did. She was pleased with herself when she was successful on the second attempt. Whilst the condoms were handled easily and with a lot of humour, it was a different story when Paul showed them a femidom. They refused to touch it or handle it. They said it looked messy and greasy, which is in fact true, but once again we were left wondering what the implications were. Was it that, for the women, the condoms are not really anything to do with them, whilst femidoms would be very much to do with them? We had vague questions about a sort of Freudian denial of female sexuality which we would want to explore further.'

The concept of sex as pleasure also appeared to be alien to some of the participants. It became clear during the course that to say No is actually very difficult. This proved unsurprising since this has much to do with lifestyle. If you are not allowed to choose your own clothes, or even to eat certain food at a particular time (many people with learning disabilities in day centres or residential homes have no control over what is provided and when), then being able to make choices about your own sexual activity is problematic. The following excerpt from the diary after participants had been to visit the Genito Urinary Clinic illustrates this clearly:

'On our way back Ms W asked Fiona all sorts of questions about sex, does it hurt, is it nice, etc. and about liking people, i.e. fancying them. It struck Fiona how little information Ms W had and that she very much needed good education about her own body, how to touch it, and how to find out what she likes and doesn't. This might be possible in

117

a group, if it were small and intimate, but Fiona thought she might benefit from one-to-one work with a female therapist.'

Much time was therefore spent in treating the subject in a straightforward but light-hearted manner which included games and fun. This was felt to be important since from the outset, many participants were nervous and embarrassed. If they were to talk to other people with learning disabilities, it was essential that they did not transmit their own nervousness or embarrassment. Hence we aimed to ensure that anxieties about sex were reduced during the course. If nothing else, this might enable participants to be more in touch with their own feelings.

A game which was particularly enjoyed was 'keeping the condom in the air'. Although a simple variant of 'keeping the balloon in the air', it enabled participants to handle condoms in a non-threatening way and also to get used to the feel of them. Another was the 'rhubarb' game where you ask a question to someone else in the group, who then answers 'rhubarb!'. The object of the game is to get the person to laugh at the question. Our variation was that each participant had to choose a word they associated with sex, such as 'bollocks'. The excerpt from the diary shows that the games were an invaluable way of lightening the atmosphere when it threatened to get heavy or oppressive;

'The games were a very successful and fun way to learn about the parts of the body, and to encourage people to say words they don't normally use, possibly even words that they are told not to use, in day centres or at home. One of the games led us to literally cry with laughter which was a wonderful release from some of the tension of the day. Lesson number one; it's useless talking at people, they don't remember what is said, what they remember is saying things for themselves, doing things and having fun.'

The group also attended both the Genito Urinary Clinic and the Family Planning Clinic. The rationale for these visits was to enable participants to know where each was and how to get there (so that they could identify the bus route and know the procedure). Photographs were taken for the portfolios to help people to recall the location. Bus routes, phone numbers and opening hours were also included in the portfolios. We found that professional staff were often unable to communicate clearly with people with learning disabilities. In addition, much of the material freely available for the general public was not accessible to people with learning disabilities as it was produced in written form. The report to Respond noted this as an issue to be addressed: 'One serious difficulty was at the GU Clinic, where there seemed to be an assumption that people with learning disabilities do not indulge in and are not subjected to different forms of sexual activity such as "rimming" or anal sex between men.'

We would certainly suggest that awareness training of professionals working in the field of sexuality and sexual health should take place with regard to learning disability and the sexual activities experienced by people with learning disabilities. We would also like to see some training around how to demystify the jargon. Some professionals, possibly embarrassed at their own prejudices, tend to use language not easily understood by lay people, including people with learning disabilities.

The diary notes also indicate that such visits need to be made part of the social training for people with learning disabilities so that they accept it as a natural event in their lives:
'Ms D struggled, but for different reasons we think. She has said that she is going to register at the clinic to go on the pill but she does not look confident or relaxed when she talks about it. In view of this we would have hoped that she would show an interest to see what to do, it seemed that in fact it was just too uncomfortable for her, and she kept out of the way as much as possible. At the Genito Urinary clinic they were interested and had no difficulty in asking the questions. At the FP clinic it seemed much harder, which may be because it feels more real to them. The clinic may well be something they need to use in their own lives now, whilst the Genito Urinary clinic is for other people'.

As the week progressed, the question of how to enlighten the participants about the nature of HIV became more pressing. Despite the visit to the Genito Urinary clinic early in the week, HIV remained a vague concept and one to be avoided at all costs. We spent much time debating whether or not this was crucial. One perspective could be that as long as people are afraid of HIV this would prevent unsafe sex. Our conclusions were that fear may be a motivating factor for a while but more importantly, people should be able to make informed decisions which, without an understanding of HIV would not be possible. This would be especially pertinent if they were to continue with the project of discussing safer sex with other people with learning disabilities.

A serious lack was a good depiction of what HIV does to the immune system. There are leaflets and books but very little has been developed with people with learning disabilities in mind. What came to mind was a demonstration, but we could not find appropriate slides or videos. We were aware that showing how HIV is contracted and how AIDS develops is difficult as the prognosis is often widely different in people with HIV and that there is no consistent course towards the onset of AIDS. There is also an on-going debate as to the nature of the virus and its origins. We decided to try and develop our own demonstration.

We experimented and we believe that we came up with a very plausible demonstration. This involved soaking a paper kitchen towel previously cut in a body shape in food colouring. The food colouring depicted the immune system. We then used a dropper to add bleach solution to a part of the body which then immediately turned white. We explained then that HIV had entered the body. It was not removable. We then added more drops and slowly more and more of the body changed into a more whitish hue from previously being dark blue. When it was almost covered in white spots, we then explained that this was likely to be AIDS as no longer could the immune system cope (Box 4).

This horrified people, as for the first time, the grim reality of AIDS struck home. While by no means perfect, we had to add more and more bleach as we went along as the paper kitchen towel material did not show any spreading - we felt that this worked excellently in showing how it happens. But the bleach smelt awful and some participants left the room. This was partly to do with the bleach but also the impact on them of better understanding HIV and AIDS, probably for the first time. The notes from the diary record our feelings at the time:

> 'The demonstration of how HIV affects the body was graphic and frightening. The atmosphere became heavy and tense. We feared at one point that we were being too explicit, by showing HIV can lead to AIDS which will lead to illness which will lead to death. We felt it would be easy to feed into the 'people with learning disabilities must be protected' syndrome and so we resisted the temptation to cover up and reassure participants. We did however show that we could see that it was scary and worrying for people.'

As with all our work, the demonstration was photographed for the portfolio. The development of the portfolio was hampered by the lack of suitable materials. We intensively used materials from the package *Sex and the 3 R's* (McCarthy & Thompson, 1992). The pictures are good in that they clearly depict different sexual positions and show a number of people which do not conform to the usual 'glossy magazine' type bodies, models or heterosexist assumptions. However, it did have one omission in that there was no picture of 'rimming'. We did not cover this activity during the course, but we did create a picture showing this in case it came up.

A surprising outcome of the portfolio work was that the participants enjoyed putting them together. The diary notes indicate that perhaps they had not been given enough opportunity to be students and given encouragement to organise their own materials:

'They were very enthusiastic about this, enjoying using the hole punch and arranging the papers. We had debated whether it would have been better to have the pages punched beforehand as it was very time consuming. However, it was agreed they would enjoy making up their own folders and it was an opportunity to either learn this skill or to practice if they had done it before. Ms D seemed particularly pleased with her folder and wanted to take it home, which she did.'

We were aware that this gathering of information might not be appreciated by carers. We therefore spent a long time discussing how best to include the carers and it was decided to write a letter with the agreement of the participants. This covered the following points.

- the participant has attended the course

- there is a folder of the work to help them to remember (and what's in it)

- they may want to talk to the carer

- outline of principles: being able to make choices, preventing unwanted pregnancy and cutting down the risk of catching HIV

- why people with learning disabilities need to learn about safer sex

- who is paying for the course and why

- that the participant may ask the carer about sex

- a contact person at Respond was identified whom carers could approach

This way of reaching the parents or carers was not altogether successful. In one case, a participant chose not to share the contents of their portfolio with her parent. Unfortunately, the parent did discover the portfolio and immediately denounced it as pornography and demanded that it be returned to Respond. In another case, the participant requested that Respond keep her portfolio in safe keeping as she felt if her mother were to see it, there would be repercussions for her.

Conclusions

The portfolio highlighted the fact that people with learning disabilities are often not considered sexual beings with opportunities for privacy in their own homes. Being unable to take home materials that are supposed to be part of your working apparatus is to our minds a denial of your potential and ability to empower yourself and others. Compiling it was constructive and enjoyable but for some, to keep it was fraught with difficulties, a sad reflection of their living situations rather than on their own attitudes towards sex.

There remains a desperate need for good quality materials with easy to read and understandable pictures. The *3 R's* goes some way to addressing this problem but is designed for teaching situations and not for information purposes which is where a great lack of competence exists. We also recommended that Respond should write to Universities as a first step towards finding a design group that could develop a clear demonstration of how HIV may develop into AIDS, in order to aid understanding of the deadliness of this virus.

Training such as this inevitably runs counter to beliefs held by many parents or to staff providing day to day support. Drastic changes in lifestyles and attitude towards empowerment and freedom of choice are needed before such training is likely to be really successful. Even within the field of education and sex training, there are those who would advocate restrictions as if people with learning disabilities are infants, powerless to make informed choices. We believe that this constitutes an infringement of liberty that should be resisted. At the same time we also need safeguards for those people who cannot make informed choices, for instance in relation to safer sex or HIV testing.

Paul chose not to use an interpreter as it was felt that this would create a barrier between the participants and himself. All but one participant learnt how to communicate face to face with him during the week. In group sessions however, particularly when difficult matters arose, the ground rules were forgotten and Paul was sometimes excluded. The dilemma between functional and emotional communication was at times impossible to resolve.

One aim was to enable people to relax when thinking and talking about sex, in order that they could start the process of discussing it with other people. Two participants decided to continue this work and talk to others. However, we feel that success is also measured by the fact that three others decided against. Not everyone wishes to be a role model. Those who do should be encouraged and empowered to do so. Training for empowerment is ultimately doomed without the full participation of those it professes to empower. People with learning disabilities, like other disadvantaged groups, require role models with whom they are able to empathise and feel confident.

We were appalled at the abusive sexual history of some of the participants and have recommended most strongly to Respond that they consider organising a course around enjoyment of sex as a process of empowerment and would wish to see this develop on a much greater scale for all sections of the population.

A further recommendation was that awareness training be set up for professionals (including the police) who often assume that people with learning disabilities do not experience sex, let alone enjoy it. We learnt from the participants that after experiencing abuse, subsequent encounters with professionals could also be abusive but in a different way.

Our final conclusion is that we can learn much in the areas of sexuality and safer sex, but this will have little impact on empowering informed choice, sexual pleasure or expression without basic issues of human rights being addressed. These are of paramount importance to the lives of most people with learning disabilities and while these are left untackled, as they are in so many services and establishments, there can be no real advancement for people with learning disabilities in living life with freedom and choices.

References

Brown, H., Stein, J. *The Sexual Abuse of Adults with Learning Disabilities: Report*
& Turk, V. (1995) *of a Second Two Year Incidence Survey*, Mental Handicap
Research, Vol.8, No.1.

McCarthy, M. & *Sex and the 3 R's - Rights, Responsibilities and Risks*, Pavilion
Thompson, D. (1992) Publishing, Brighton.

Probert, R. (1973) in The Penguin Dictionary of Modern Humorous Quotations,
Compiled by Fred Metcalf, Guild Publishing 1989.

Fiona Barber holds a CQSW and is currently working as a transitions social worker for the London borough of Wandsworth. She has several years experience working with people with learning disabilities in residential and educational settings, having facilitated 'parents' and 'friendship skills' groups. Her association with Respond included membership of the Management Committee, involvement with the 1993 conference and chairing the 1994 conference 'From Denial to Justice'.

Paul Redfern is a writer and tutor and is now working as a partner of Deafworks, a deaf-led company employing deaf tutors, graphic designers, illustrators and office staff. He has edited the Deafview pages for Teletext and presented the Tyne Tees TV 'Sign On' and the BBC 'See Hear!' programmes. He has also edited the Council on Deafness newsletter. Paul holds workshops for deaf people to improve their teaching of British Sign Language after teaching BSL to hearing students.

Chapter 9

Sex Education for Students
with Severe Learning Disabilities

by David Stewart

'I shall the effect of this good lesson keep as watchman to my heart.'
Thus does Ophelia respond to advice on conducting relationships.

Background

The counselling of young people on the subject of sex and relationships still amazingly remains an activity which causes angst for adults and young people alike and dilemmas for those providing support and advice. When young people also have learning disabilities, the situation appears to go from bad to worse. Further taboos come into play, with rights ignored and sexuality denied. This chapter sets out to explore how one school has attempted to address the issue of sex and relationship education with students and pupils with severe learning disabilities. It is important at this point to remember the duty of all governing bodies to have a sex education policy. Recent legislation (Sex Education Act,1993) has been less than helpful to all age special schools who find themselves with the possibility of an optional policy for the primary department and a compulsory one for those of secondary age. The important factor however, is that the subject is now officially on the agenda, although the potential of such policies has been tempered by exclusion at the individual level. It has now been some time since parents were given the right to opt their child out of sex education at school. To date, no such request has been made at Shepherd School. We are also fortunate in having an education authority which has a written policy on sex education for all students *and* one which directly addresses the needs of students with special needs.

The Shepherd School in Nottingham, is a large day school for pupils and students with severe learning disabilities aged between 3 and 19. In total there are some 160 pupils. In the early eighties some concern was expressed that sex education, for various reasons, was not being tackled as part of school policy, even though students were facing situations with which they needed guidance.

We were asked by parents for advice on masturbation, menstruation or other sexual behaviours and by police and social workers about our policy on sex education. Students found themselves in trouble for inappropriate behaviour and yet there had been little inputs to guide them or their carers. Some staff recognised the need for effective sex education, while others hoped to ignore it and felt it could be appropriately dealt with by adult services, as though nothing significant happened until 19! Clearly the attitude and reactive practice, represented by the comment 'we deal with matters when they arise', was of little help in developing any longer term strategy (it is alarming that this 'emergency first aid' approach is still too prevalent in special schools). There are as yet few examples of good practice in sex education for young people with severe learning disabilities who attend mainstream schools.

Establishing the Initiative

Some 10 years ago discussion was instigated amongst staff. There are nearly 90 staff, both teaching and non-teaching and consequently some 90 opinions on the subject. They ranged from 'sex only happens in marriage and as most students will not marry there is no need to bother', to 'they should do what they want when they want'. One member of staff was even of the opinion that boys 'don't masturbate', another that her pupils were too young. It is important to encourage discussion and yet focus it on producing and raising awareness and sensitivity. Staff concerns only reflect the concerns of parents and society in general. We continue to seek a middle road with which staff feel comfortable, but become aware of avoidance tactics. The most important thing is to provide a forum where people can be honest about their feelings and concerns about the whole area of sexuality, including the sexuality of young people.

Some staff are likely to feel uncomfortable about teaching certain areas of the sex education programme. That can be accepted up to a point, but no staff member can avoid being confronted with questions, situations or inappropriate behaviours or exempted from giving considered and consistent responses. The way staff approach such situations is all part of 'sex education' and without due thought can cause distress and damage. At the same time, staff need continual support and training to gain confidence. It is interesting to note that central Government provides no direct training budget for non-teaching staff, despite their daily interactions with staff and students.

There also needs to be much sensitivity when working with staff whose only experience of working with children with learning disabilities has been in one context, whether at a certain establishment or in their own local community, as experience and horizons may be limited. It is consequently essential to take a great deal of time and there will be the need for continuing education for everyone. All kinds of doubts, prejudices and fears will be encountered, and those with the ultimate responsibility for ensuring that the sex education curriculum is delivered will need to be robust and resiliant to support not only themselves but their colleagues.

Consultation and Direction

Advice was sought from others as to the best approach. It was suggested that we set up a monitoring group which would not only monitor the programme but would also act as a buffer between the school and the wider community in the event of any criticism (although there has been none). Staff need to feel supported in this sensitive area and approaches were made to people who were felt to understand our needs. As sex education is the responsibility of the governors (in England and Wales) it was important to establish the Chairman of Governors, who is also a social worker, as chair of the group. The school representatives include three other governors, one of whom is also a parent, the head teacher, and school staff representatives. Representatives of the wider community include a local JP, the community policeman, the school nurse, a retired health promotion manager, an educational psychologist, a chaplain and Dr Ann Craft of the Department of Learning Difficulties at Nottingham University.

The group not only vets the materials and programmes to be used but also monitors lessons in school and the effectiveness of programmes. This puts teachers on the line, but has proved beneficial, as observers are able to comment on the relevance of the materials used and the techniques adopted. This is fed back and acted upon. For instance, a teacher may be discussing the practicalities of dealing with periods with a group of female students. She may be giving one message verbally but her body language is saying something different and this is confusing for students.

The group has also given a priority to liaison with parents and carers through workshops and meetings. In the initial phase all parents were given a copy of the school policy and programme for sex education. Meetings were arranged to enable the policy to be discussed and to show educational materials.

127

These provided an opportunity for parents to express their wish for further workshops on specific topics such as masturbation and menstruation. The group was concerned to work *alongside* parents, so as not to provide an 'expert' perspective, allowing discussion of problems and sharing ideas for dealing with them. These meetings proved very successful. The workshops included the topics of masturbation, menstruation, the needs of those with profound and multiple learning disabilities, HIV and AIDS, the use of public toilets for sex and personal protection in an abuse and sexual health context. Workshops dealing with abuse were very well attended and some useful discussion occurred. I feel that this was because previous meetings had established a vocabulary for meaningful dialogue. Parents now feel able to discuss issues which might have previously caused embarrassment.

Parents' Meetings

Working with parents on such sensitive areas is likely to appear daunting at first but confidence is gained with experience. I even recall a meeting when no parents turned up, illustrating the need for perseverance. The monitoring group has been keen to ensure that parents feel some ownership of the meetings. In the early days the meetings attracted few parents of younger children They no doubt thought the issues were not relevant to them. However, parents who were experiencing difficulties or uncertainties with young people in their teens were quick to disabuse these parents, pointing out their missed opportunity to consider this important area of their child's life. Parents are kept up to date with any new materials and members of the monitoring group are able to report what they have seen in class.

As an outcome of the meetings we produced some simple booklets intended to help parents. They are entirely based on what parents discussed at the meetings and therefore reflect common concerns and anxieties. Some parents come to a group and are unable to communicate their concerns or unwilling to share what they have learnt with other family members. The booklets have acted as a useful reference aid and a reminder of the issues involved. They cover the issues of menstruation, masturbation for boys, masturbation for girls, HIV and AIDS, personal protection, sexuality and profound and multiple learning disabilities. These booklets are now widely used throughout the UK. It is important that people working on these issues share information and exchange their experiences of what may be of use to young people and their carers. It is essential that there is a balance between the use of articles in learned journals aimed at professionals and the availability of good clear advice to as many people as possible. We are also able to share with parents the fact that staff also have very real apprehensions. For example, some male members of staff expressed concerns about the subject of sexual abuse. Staff in special schools are sometimes in situations involving personal care such as genital hygiene or learning how to use a urinal or how to shower, teaching self care skills their colleagues in mainstream education would not have to address. There clearly need to be guidelines and procedures to protect students and staff.

There are no easy solutions but it is important to keep the matter to the fore in discussion. The father who may be the only person who can lift his multiple disabled daughter into the bath may have very similar concerns and anxieties. Other management issues are raised by the fact that the majority of staff are female and may well be involved in the care of teenage boys. How appropriate are these considerations when we try to encourage privacy and respect? Some female staff said they didn't mind but we also have to ask whether young men really want this. Others might argue that it is preferable to have a mixture of male and female staff in the care of male students. There was clearly plenty of scope for further debate.

Curriculum Development

Clearly, sex education cannot be divorced from other areas of health and relationship education and the Document 5 (NCC, 1990) sets it very much on the agenda as part of the National Curriculum. I feel strongly that sex education must be set out as a discrete area as there is a danger that it can get lost in a general programme: students could spend a great deal of time learning how to wash their hands and faces without tackling the more sensitive area of health education. Students need to start such education early and it is too late to start when the young person enters puberty. A useful vocabulary needs to be established. All too often students have no names for parts of the body and owing to their isolation from their peers they do not even have a vocabulary of slang words. They often therefore have little concept of their body and consequently it is difficult to establish good self awareness and self esteem.

If you mention sex education at the nursery you will usually be met by a shocked response, but what are we really talking about here? I have already said that it is important that children know about and value their bodies. As important is the establishment of skills of choice and decision making. When are young children allowed to make a choice? Does a child at the nursery get the opportunity to choose between an Apple or an Orange? Are they allowed to wear the T-shirt they like best. If these skills are not established early, they are certainly not going to learn about sex overnight at the age of 16 when parents and staff might suddenly become aware of their vulnerability. The fact that certain behaviour patterns are set when students are very young means that work needs to start early. Children who are allowed to kiss and cuddle with anyone indiscriminately are not only wide open to possible abuse, they also render themselves socially unacceptable. Too often adults allow such behaviour either because they don't want to hurt feelings or because they themselves have a need to be loved. We must always question whose need is being met and why different standards are being set for people with learning disabilities.

It is important that education should seek to establish a feeling of self worth, help students to live more satisfying lives and give them skills to have more control over their lives. The programme should give knowledge and information about the physical self. This will need to be updated as students develop, as what is taught about the body at the age of eight needs expansion when entering puberty. This highlights the need for a spiral curriculum. It is important to encourage an exploration and understanding of feelings and emotions. Students need to look at values and examine appropriate behaviours. Opportunities for decision making and self advocacy clearly also need to be on the agenda.

Friendships and Relationships

Opportunities for establishing friendships and relationships are extremely difficult for students with severe learning disabilities. We attach great importance to friendship, but how are friendships and relationships allowed to develop? Is it vital that we work closely with the students and their families to promote these opportunities? And what is a friend? All too often the circle of people with whom our young people enjoy social time and social contact are paid workers which creates an unnatural situation for the development of relationships.

Simply meeting somebody for the first time does not mean they will become a friend or make them a potential sexual partner. In a school or other institutional setting it is very difficult for young people to express and develop more intimate friendships, associations or other relationships. Families, parents and other carers therefore need to give this whole area very careful consideration. Young people with severe learning disabilities become isolated from their peers. They are unlikely to have access to transport or other means of communication with friends. They come to school, work, have recreational time and carry out their relationships and interactions all under the eyes of staff. When we discuss relationships we cannot ignore marriage or cohabitation and the considerations for two people living together. For some people, parenthood will also be on the agenda. Students will for instance, notice the attention given to family members who marry and have children. They will also note the social status that having a partner brings, yet the vast majority of people with learning disabilities will never have a satisfying relationship or have children, which gives people direct messages about their worth in society. A great deal of work needs to be done to value people in their own right. One can be single, happy, have friends, play a useful role in society and be awarded worth. Families need to support this notion rather than give mixed messages by humouring supposed 'crushes' but not allowing the development of true relationships.

Longer Term Initiatives

For a year, an officer from the health authority worked with senior students on the subject of HIV and AIDS. Most of the time was spent on establishing what a friend is. It became very apparent that unless this was established much of the other work became meaningless. I think it also highlights that there needs to be long term planning and acceptance that such work should be ongoing. Education on sex and relationships and sexual health is never completed and you can never say the student knows everything. It is easy to forget that students with severe learning difficulties are no different.

In 1988 the school became involved in a project with Ann Craft to write a programme of sex education for people with learning disabilities. With other schools, further education colleges and adult centres, a programme was devised and trialled by other establishments around the country (Craft, 1991). The programme, entitled *Living Your Life*, covers all areas of sex and relationship education and is accompanied by visual aids. The school was also involved in a Nottinghamshire County Council project on child protection from 1987 to 1989. From that project, books were produced which took simple plots based around possible abusive behaviour. They are accompanied by Makaton symbols. There are also simple games for young pupils, devised to look at different situations and establish the element of choice and decision making which is essential if students are to protect themselves (LDA, 1994).

131

Sexual Abuse

The acknowledgement of abuse, particularly that of people with severe learning disabilities was a long time coming and denial and disbelief are still encountered. The work of NAPSAC (National Association for the Protection from Sexual Abuse of Adults and Children with Learning Disabilities) including through its newsletter and of the organisation Voice, has done much to raise people's awareness. Skills which need to be taught and targeted are assertiveness, decision making, choice and general communication. A long role play programme can be a most effective method, but here too, rules and skills will need to be learnt. A most useful resource in the use of role play and drama is *On the Agenda* (Image In Action, 1994).

Defining and identifying abuse is difficult. It is very difficult if you do not value yourself or your body in particular. Deprived of physical affection or touch as a young adult, what might you permit for the sake of physical warmth or closeness. What if you like what is happening to you? There has been a tendency for some parents to see sterilisation or the pill as some universal panacea to managing the most immediate consequences of sexual activity. Such responses do not prevent sexual abuse, rape, HIV or other sexually transmitted infections, nor do they reflect the range of sex, including homosexuality, experienced by people with learning disabilities. The danger is that carers think they no longer need to worry or indeed to provide education. Work also has to be done with some older students to ensure that they understand that some of their behaviours might also be perceived as abusive. The only person who will play with a teenage person with learning disabilities is often a five year old child. The parent of that child may see the young person as a possible abuser, so considerable counselling may be needed.

HIV

It is essential that students and families are made aware of the need for education in HIV. There has been a tendency in the past to consider that people with learning disabilities are not affected. There is a need to disabuse people of this idea, as young people with learning disabilities are particularly vulnerable because of society's attitude to students having relationships. For instance, students may have quick and furtive sex at the back of a centre. How is a condom to be obtained and safer sex negotiated?

What messages do we give out to young people about sexuality? Schools, unlike adult centres, are not bound by clause 28, yet there is still confusion about the discussion of same sex relationships. There is a tendency to assume that all young peoples' relationships or sexual encounters will be heterosexual. Yet we know from colleagues in the adult sector that there will be situations and opportunities for same sex activity. If for instance we have taught young men that they should wear a condom when having penetrative vaginal sex with a woman, will they think that its OK not to use a condom when having penetrative anal sex with a man! Terms like 'partner' may mean little to someone with a learning disability. We need to spell things out clearly and students need to be prepared for the real world, not one which society thinks they will encounter. Authorities, managers and parents need to think this reality through very carefully and respond to it.

During workshops on HIV and AIDS, parents and carers expressed ignorance of many of the facts about transmission and have welcomed the education as much for themselves as for their young people. There remains considerable ignorance and uncertainty about such questions in the population at large, and we must work together to provide support and information. It is difficult for parents to think their children may be open to abuse or may engage in same sex relationships and very sensitive work may be required. To deny this work is to negate the very messages we are striving to give about valuing and appreciating body and mind.

Human resources are also important. We have established links with our local GUM clinic and staff there are very willing to talk to students and show them around. They explain the procedures and allay any fears the students may have. In Nottingham we also have a Health Shop where anyone can go for advice and our students are made familiar with this resource. Until recently there was also a Well Woman Clinic for women with learning disabilities. This was a valuable resource which needs to re-open.

Using Resources

At this point it may prove useful to identify and discuss those resources which we have found most useful. This is clearly not an exhaustive list and resources need to be under constant review. When choosing appropriate material we initially found the resources of the Health Education Unit very useful. Clearly such sources reflect an interest in this area by the unit and its usefulness has changed over the years. Other establishments have always been invaluable in exchanging ideas and observations about particular resources. Boxes 1, 2 and 3 summarise the resources we have used for work with staff, parents and students respectively.

133

Box I
WORK WITH STAFF

Options for Change (Dixon, 1986).
Sex and Staff Training (McCarthy & Thompson, 1994).
Disability Equality in the Classroom, A Human Rights Issue (Reiser & Mann, 1992).
Religion, Ethnicity And Sex Education (NCB, 1993).
Disable Discrimination (Baxter, 1990).
Special Health (Craft & Combes, 1989).
It Could Never Happen Here (ARC/NAPSAC, 1993).
The Chailey Heritage guidelines(Chailey Heritage, 1992).
The ABCD Pack (NSPCC, 1993)
'kids scope programme for special needs' (Hitchen, 1992)

Box 2
WORK WITH PARENTS

Work with parents has been documented in Parental Involvement, in the sex education of students with severe learning disabilities (Croft & Cromby, 1991). At Shepherd School we have six booklets previously described for use by parents. These are available from the school. What About Us! (Craft & Stewart, 1993) is a text aimed at parents and staff.

Box 3
WORK WITH STUDENTS

Student schemes include Living Your Life (Craft, 1991). Chance To Choose (Dixon, 1994). Sex and the 3R's (McCarthy & Thompson, 1993). Not a Child Anymore (Brook Advisory, 1989) has particularly good visual resources. Models are very useful, particularly with students who find photographs or line drawings difficult to comprehend.

There is still much to develop in the field of sexuality and students with particular multiple learning disabilities. Current projects at Nottingham University should yield much. At present there is the booklet from The Shepherd School series which addresses this area for parents. *Planning a Multisensory Massage Programme for Very Special People* (Longhorn, 1993) may well provide some useful practice for staff.

Conclusion

As a school I think we have increased our competence of supporting sexuality in all areas of the school community and improved our practice with students, better addressing their needs. There is still much to be done and it is a continuing story, as students move on, new parents come on to the scene and staff change. Our views of understanding of society and sexuality also change. There is need for ongoing discussion, time for reflection and much need for training. We are fortunate in having supportive governors, a sympathetic education committee and parents who are rising to the challenge. Some people argue that much of this cannot be relevant to our students but who is to say what experiences they will meet in life. They have a right to lead safe and satisfying lives, making as much choice as possible. Sex may not be compulsory, but sex education is.

NAPSAC's address
Floor E
South Block
University Hospital
Nottingham
NG7 2UH

VOICE's address
PO Box 238
Derby
DE1 9JN

Chapter 9

References

ARC/NAPSAC (1993) *It Could Never Happen Here*, Association for Residential Care/National Association for the Protection from Sexual Abuse of Adults and Children with Learning Disabilities, Nottingham

Baxter, C. (1990) *Disable Discrimination*, King's Fund Centre, London.

Brook Advisory (1989) *Not a Child Anymore,* Brook Advisory, London.

Chailey Heritage (1992) *Chailey Heritage Guidelines,* Child Protection Policies and Procedures for Disabled Children in Residential Care, Chailey Heritage, Sussex.

Craft, A. (1991) *Living your Life*, LDA, Wisbech.

Craft, A. & Combes, (1989) *Special Health,* Health Education Authority, London.

Craft, A. & Stewart, D. (1993) *What About Us!* Home and School Council, Sheffield.

Craft, A. & Cromby, J. (1991) *Parental Involvement,* Department of Learning Disability, University of Nottingham.

Dixon, H. (1986) *Options for Change in the Sex Education of Students with severe learning difficulties*, Family Planning Association, London.

Dixon, H. (1994) *Chance to Choose,* LDA, Wisbech.

Hitchen, M. (1992) *Kidscape Programme adapted for pupils with learning difficulties*, Pringle School, Staffordshire.

Image in Action (1994) *On the Agenda,* Image in Action, London.

LDA (1994) *The Protection Pack*, LDA, Wisbech.

Longhorn, F. (1993) *Planning a Multi-sensory Massage Programme for very Special People,* Orcha Services, London.

McCarthy, M. &   *Sex and the 3 Rs*, Pavilion, Brighton.
Thompson, D. (1992)

McCarthy, M. &   *Sex and Staff Training*, Pavilion, Brighton.
Thompson, D. (1994)

NCB (1993)   *Religion, Ethnicity and Sex Education*, National Children's
                       Bureau.

NCC (1990)   *Document No.5, 'Health Education'*, National Curriculum
                       Council, London.

NSPCC (1993)   *ABCD Pack*, National Society for the Prevention of Cruelty to
                       Children, Leicester.

NCCE (1993)   *Curriculum Guidelines for Sex Education in Notts Schools,
                       'Sex Education in Special Schools'*, Nottinghamshire County
                       Council Education Department, Nottingham.

Reiser, M. &   *Disability Equality in the Classroom; a Human Rights Issue*
Manson, M. (1992)   Disability Equality in Education, London.

Stewart, D   *Now They are Growing Up*, Shepherd School, Nottingham.
(1990-1996)

The '*Now They are Growing Up*' series includes:
1. Masturbation - male
2. Masturbation - female
3. Menstruation
4. A planned dependent life and sexuality
5. Protecting your child
6. HIV and AIDS
(Nos. 1,2,3 and 5 also in Punjabi and Urdu).

David Shepherd is the Head of the Shepherd School for pupils and students with severe learning disabilities, Nottingham. For many years he was the co-ordinator of the school's sex education monitoring group. He has published 'What About Us' with Ann Craft, and was editor of the 'Protection Pack'. The school was much involved with the development of 'Living Your Life'. David has a particular interest in the arts and disability.

Chapter 10

The Law, HIV and People with Learning Disabilities

by Michael Gunn

There are a number of specific legal issues which are of potential concern to services for people with learning disabilities, support workers and advocates in relation to people with learning disabilities and HIV infection and AIDS. First, there is the question of testing for the presence of the HIV virus. Second, there is the question of possible liability for causing an HIV positive status in another person. Third, there is the question of providing information to others about the HIV status of a person with learning disabilities. Finally, there is the possibility of the 'AIDS legislation' being used in relation to a person with learning disabilities. The aim of this chapter is to address all four questions.

HIV Testing

1. The law of battery and assault
Where it has been decided to take an HIV test because it is suspected that a person may have HIV infection, the essential requirement is that the consent of that person should be obtained. Without consent, the taking of a blood sample would involve both a battery and an assault, each of which are crimes and civil wrongs. The consent given to the bodily contact involved in the taking of the sample prevents the commission of a crime or a civil wrong. It is probably not the case that failure to provide information as to the usage to which the sample was to be put would make the taking of the blood sample a battery and therefore unlawful.

2. The law of negligence: information provision
The taking of the sample would be negligent where insufficient information was provided to the person prior to its taking. It appears to be good practice to provide a person from whom a sample is to be taken with information about what is to happen to that sample (Roth & Gryk, 1995). Good practice is likely also to be a legal requirement, as the standards of the relevant medical profession are likely, as a consequence, to demand that information

be provided prior to the taking of a sample (*Sidaway v Bethiem*, Royal Hospital, 1984). If the information is not provided and the person would not have had the sample taken had the information been provided, the civil wrong (or tort) of negligence has been committed.

3. Competence and learning disability
The fact that the person from whom a sample is to be taken is a person with learning disabilities makes no necessary difference to the legal position. However, there are some issues to be noted. The first potential difference arises when considering whether the person with learning disabilities concerned is *able* to provide the consent in order to prevent the commission of a battery or assault (for further information see Gunn, 1994 and for proposals for reform of the law, Gunn, 1995). The competency of the person to make the decision whether to have the sample taken must be determined. There are three possible tests for competency which are different in their details. The one most likely to be demanded by the law is that developed by Thorpe in *Re C*, (1993). Thorpe took the view that the essential question was to ask whether 'Mr C. 's capacity is so reduced by his chronic mental illness that he does not sufficiently understand the nature, purpose and effects of the proffered amputation.' In determining whether this test is satisfied, Thorpe accepted that the approach propounded by Eastman, when giving expert evidence in the case, was helpful. Dr. Eastman suggested that the decision making process may be divided into three stages

(i)   the individual must comprehend and retain treatment information

(ii)   the individual must believe the information with which he or she is supplied, and

(iii) the individual must weigh that information in the balance to arrive at a choice as to whether to accept the treatment.

It is arguable that this sets a higher standard for an individual to comply with than the 'broad terms' approach which may be derived from the judgement of Bristow in *Chatterton v Gerson* (1981). That approach appeared to demand merely that the individual had to understand the broad terms of the treatment. However, the test in *Re C* appears to be the correct test, as it is more recent, the issue was central to the decision in the case, and it is more consistent with the approach to competence propounded in paragraph 15.10 of the Mental Health Act Code of Practice (1993), which states:

'An individual in order to have capacity must be able to:

- *understand what medical treatment is and that somebody has said that he needs it and why the treatment is being proposed;*

- *understand in broad terms the nature of the proposed treatment;*

- *understand its principal benefits and risks;*

- *understand what will be the consequences of not receiving the proposed treatment;*

- *possess the capacity to make a choice.'*

If the person has the capacity to make the decision, it may need to be established that he or she did actually have that capacity and did make a choice at the time a decision was needed. The difference between having the capacity to make a decision and actually making that decision is not valid in the context of the general law with regard to decision-making and so the distinction drawn by Mr. Justice Stuart-Smith in *R v Mental Health Act Commission, ex parte X* (1988) is to be regarded as relevant only to an interpretation of the Mental Health Act 1983.

If a person with learning disabilities is competent to make the decision whether to have the sample taken, the decision is solely for him or her to take, provided that he or she is an adult. If a person is not competent to make that decision, the law allows for steps to be taken, provided they fall within the criteria established in *Re F* (1990) - (for further information see Morgan, 1990; Gunn, 1990; Gunn, 1996). It would have to be established that the taking of a blood sample in order to test for HIV was in the best interests of the individual from whom the sample was to be taken. Taking a sample for testing because of *staff* concerns is not sufficient. In *Re F* the concept of best interests was interpreted as meaning what was consistent with the standards of a responsible body of medical opinion; a strange way of approaching the concept (Morgan, 1990). Nevertheless, the primary focus is on the benefit which accrues to the person with learning disabilities from having the test and which would most obviously be satisfied by tying in the results of the test with the provision of appropriate care and treatment.

4.   Issues associated with testing
Two difficult issues associated with having a test for HIV arise. These are concerned with the consequences which might flow from having a test. First, consequences flowing from the simple fact of having the test, and second, the

consequences where there is an HIV positive result.

At one time it was the case that life assurance companies demanded that prospective insured persons had to declare whether they had had a test for HIV and whether they had received counselling for AIDS. Since the contract of insurance is one of 'uberrimae fides', that is of the utmost good faith, failure to provide that information destroyed the basis of the contract and so the individual's insurance was completely invalid (Roth & Gryk, 1995, pp.90-91). However, the Association of British Insurers recently announced a new Statement of Practice entitled 'Underwriting Life Insurance for HIV/AIDS' in July 1994. Adoption of that Statement will mean that insurance companies will not ask whether someone has tested for HIV but whether they have had a positive test and they will also not ask whether the proposer has received counselling for AIDS (Roth & Gryk, 1995, p.91). It is still the case that searching questions which seek to elicit the risk status of the individual are asked (Roth & Gryk, 1995), but those concerns are not directly relevant to the issue in hand.

Where a positive HIV rest result is provided, it might be the case that continuing a sexual relationship or starting a new one might involve criminal liability. Before considering that possibility, it might be the case that, where the person who is known to be HIV positive has a learning disability, others may be responsible for that individual's behaviour, perhaps giving rise to civil liability to anyone harmed as a consequence. The law is not keen on imposing liability on one person for the actions of a third party which have caused harm to another. However, where the third party is not to be regarded as fully responsible for her or his actions, the issue of liability might more easily arise.

Some people with learning disabilities in the care of others might well be regarded as falling into such a category, particularly if they are either known to be HIV positive or if there is an identifiable risk of them being infected with HIV. It is therefore possible, that if the person with learning disabilities infects another person with HIV through sexual intercourse, the carers or support worker might be legally responsible where the partner gets the infection (and hence their employers through vicarious liability). It would have to be proved by the person infected (or by someone on their behalf if not capable of pursuing litigation themselves, which may be the case with a person with learning disability) that the staff or carer could reasonably have foreseen this harm either because the person infected was known to be HIV positive or at risk of HIV infection, known to be engaging in a sexual relationship with the person with learning disabilities or because he or she was in a relatively small and/or obvious group of people with whom the person with learning disabilities might consort. It would then have to be shown that the carer or support worker did not take appropriate action to prevent the spread of HIV infection.

There is however only limited action that can be taken. Where a person is not detained under the Mental Health Act 1983 or the Public Health (Control of Diseases) Act 1984, there is limited control over a person's freedom of movement which may be exercised. Endeavouring to control the freedom of movement for the benefit of the individual may be justifiable in some limited circumstances, as outlined in the Mental Health Act Code of Practice (1993, paras. 18.24-18.27), but restricting freedom on the off-chance of spreading HIV-infection would not seem to be sufficient to warrant keeping a person in a particular environment. Clearly, action is appropriate and would be required to educate the person who has a learning disability, and who has (or is at risk of having) HIV infection, about his or her responsibilities, the inappropriateness of engaging in unsafe or even safer sex without the other person knowing of his or her actual or possible HIV status, and the possibility of criminal liability where he or she does have sex (for further information see Gunn, 1996).

Finally, even if the carer or support worker were in breach of his or her duty to others for failing to watch over the person with learning disabilities, it would still be necessary for the person harmed to prove that it was that breach that caused the harm, therefore there would be a real difficulty where the person harmed was more widely sexually active or at HIV risk or there was nothing that the carer or support worker could have lawfully done to prevent the spread of HIV infection.

Criminal Liability for the Spread of HIV Infection

The HIV status of a sexual partner may be a matter of real concern. If both parties are aware of the HIV positive status of one, continuing sexual activity appears not to be likely to involve the commission of an offence, and is a matter solely for the individuals to determine. However, where the HIV positive status of one person is known to one and unknown to the other it might well appear that the person with HIV should be under a legal obligation to inform the partner. Further, many would suggest that if a person who knows that he or she has HIV deliberately does not inform the partner, a criminal offence is committed by him or her. In fact, there is a technically very difficult argument involved here, as it might be also assumed that rape is committed.

Rape involves a man having sexual intercourse (vaginal or anal) with a woman or a man who does not consent to the sex. If the man knows he has HIV, it might be thought that the man or woman may only consent if they know of that status. The 19th century case of *R v Clarence* (1888), however, creates a significant problem. The husband had gonorrhoea and did not tell his wife, who had sexual intercourse with him. It was held that he was not guilty of rape, in part because of the old rule that a man could not be found guilty of rape when he had non-consensual sex with his wife. That rule has now gone, but the case also stands for the proposition that the consent of the woman (and also now a man) is only invalid where the fraud of the man causes her (or him) not to know the nature and quality of the act. If therefore, she believes that he is performing an operation to improve her singing, whereas in fact he is having sexual intercourse with her, she is mistaken as to the nature and quality of the act, and her apparent consent is not valid. However, where a woman has sexual intercourse with a diseased man, the basic act is still sexual intercourse and so there is no mistake as to the nature and quality of the act.

Ormerod and Gunn (1996) have argued, first that *Clarence* is a case which should be overruled as it creates a rule which is no longer acceptable. This is not an argument likely to succeed, as the rule has existed for so long, that the courts would more likely look to Parliament as being the appropriate forum for change. Second, they argued that *Clarence* is distinguishable since, where the man knows he has HIV, the disease is life threatening and so the nature and quality of the act are indeed different, that is sex with a man with a life-threatening condition is different in nature and quality from sex with a healthy man or a man with a non-life threatening disease. If this analysis is correct, then rape may be committed where a man who knows he has HIV and has sex with a woman or man who, though apparently consenting, would not have consented if they had known of his condition, and he is aware that they would not have so consented.

A similar argument might apply to a woman (who knows that she has HIV) having sexual intercourse with a man or a woman. The sexual offences legislation assumes that only men have sexual intercourse,

144

therefore the relevant offence where a woman is considered to be the offending party is that of indecent assault. Provided the woman takes an active
part in the sexual intercourse she will commit an assault on the man or woman
which, in the circumstances under consideration, will be indecent (for
discussion of this offence in a different context see later section).
However, the same obstacle to conviction of the woman is presented as
considered above, which is that surrounding the consent of her sexual
partner. If the arguments propounded above operate to secure the conviction of a man, so also ought they operate to secure the conviction of a woman
for indecent assault.

In fact, Ormerod and Gunn identify the commission of another offence, that
is the administration of a noxious substance contrary to section 23 or 24
of the Offences Against the Person Act 1861. Here the argument is that in
all vaginal or seminal fluids the virus is present, so it is administered by way
of completed sexual intercourse. The HIV virus is a noxious substance
because it has fatal consequences. The consent of the woman (or man) to the
sexual intercourse is either made irrelevant by the argument about *Clarence*
or the consent only extends to sex and not the administration of a noxious
substance. It is submitted that this offence could also apply to a woman,
although there might be greater problems in establishing that the substance was
administered.

If the person who knowingly risks transmitting HIV is a person with learning
disability, there is therefore a risk of criminal liability. However, these
offences require 'mens rea', which demands in these contexts, that the
person either intends to produce the consequence or is reckless (in the
sense that he or she realises the risk and nevertheless takes it). It is possible,
therefore, that a particular individual might not have the requisite foresight
and so not be deemed guilty.

It is, of course, not always the case that a person will know they have HIV.
However, they may be aware of a (high) risk. It would seem that the arguments
propounded with regard to the offences of rape and indecent assault could
not then work, or at least it would be even harder to secure a conviction of a
man or woman having unprotected sex not knowing they have HIV, but realising
that there is a (high) risk that he or she is HIV positive. If the charge were
of some other offence, such as that of administering a noxious substance contrary
to section 23 or 24 of the Offences against the Person Act 1861 then it can be

145

argued that a conviction is possible, since being reckless as to status may amount to the sufficient mental element for the commission of the offence. It is clear that the individual defendant must foresee the risk of administering the virus.

Sex and Learning Disability

If the sexual partner is a person with learning disability, the law is not necessarily different. The same law in general, applies to all people whether or not they have learning disabilities. The question of whether the person is capable of consenting to sexual intercourse may well arise. It would have to be established whether a person understood broadly what was involved in sexual intercourse. There is no clear law on this point, so it is unclear whether any more needs be understood than it is an act in which adults may engage if they wish. It may be that some knowledge of the connection between sexual intercourse and pregnancy is required. By analogy with the nature and quality of the act argument above, it seems likely that some but not much understanding of the consequences of sexual intercourse is required. I would suggest that a person cannot be competent unless, at least, he or she realises that the woman may become pregnant as a consequence of heterosexual intercourse.

If a person has a severe learning difficulty, there are specific laws which apply, but only if they fall within the definition of a 'defective' in the Sexual Offences Act 1956 or 'severe mental handicap' in the Sexual Offences Act 1967 (for further information see Gunn, 1996). The two terms have the same definition, which means that the terms refer to:

'a person suffering from a state of arrested or incomplete development of mind which includes severe impairment of intelligence and social functioning.'

This definition has three elements, each of which must be satisfied:

(i) The person must have a state of arrested or incomplete development of mind which includes people whose mind does not fully develop because of genetic causes or problems at birth causing brain damage or problems caused in the early years of life so that the mind development which was occurring is not completed. It would seem to exclude brain damage caused once the mind has developed.

(ii) A guide to the severe impairment of intelligence is that the person's I.Q. is below 50. Whilst such a result would not be taken in isolation to determine the question, it is likely to be a significant factor.

(iii) A person's social functioning would seem to refer to their ability to look after themselves and to relate with others. Adaptive behaviour test results may be of some assistance provided that the issue is identified as being the satisfaction of the statutory definition and not merely the outcome of the tests. The more socially capable the individual the less likely that he or she is a 'defective' however low her or his intelligence.

It is an offence for a man to have unlawful sexual intercourse with a woman who is severely learning disabled. This offence is committed even if the woman apparently consents, because consent is not a defence. If the couple are married, the sexual intercourse is not unlawful and so no offence is committed (see Gunn, 1996, section 3.4). There is also a statutory defence whereby the man is not guilty if he did not know and had no reason to suspect that the woman was severely learning disabled (See Gunn, 1996, section 3.9).

It is also an offence for a man or a woman indecently to assault a person who has severe learning disabilities (see Gunn, 1996, section 3.9). This means that any sexual activity involves an offence. The activity must involve actual contact or contact must be apprehended by the 'victim', therefore films do not involve the commission of this offence. A person who has severe learning disabilities is not in law, able to consent but teaching personal hygiene and any teaching involving contact or apprehended contact which is required for the person with learning disabilities to understand the implications of HIV status would not be thought indecent, therefore no offence would be committed. It is important that it be recognised that this offence imposes potential limits, not only on sexual activity in which a person who has severe learning disabilities may engage, but also on the types of non-abstract, hands-on teaching methods which may be used in sex and safer sex education programmes. If the activity can be viewed as being decent, no offence is committed, even where the person to whom the service is being offered is not allowed by law, to provide consent (Gunn, 1996, section 3.11).

A man who has a severe learning disability may not provide consent so as to make lawful what would otherwise be a homosexual offence (see Gunn, 1996, section 3.10). Homosexual offences include the offence of gross indecency and buggery. Homosexual offences are lawful (provided also that there is consent) where the act takes place in 'private' (see Gunn, 1996, section 3.10). However, a man who is has severe learning disabilities may, inconsistently with what has just been said, provide consent to what would otherwise be

147

rape: which can now be committed on a man as well as a woman (for further information see Card, 1995 and Gunn, 1996, section 3.10).

Carer's Criminal Liability

In the previous two sections, the criminal liability of a person with HIV has been considered. As a general rule others who participate in the commission of an offence by that person, who would be known, technically, as the principal offender, are also guilty of the offence committed by that principal. Others participate if they *aid, abet, counsel or procure*, which in brief, requires them to help, assist or produce the commission of the offence. But such secondary participants will only be liable where they intend to help or encourage, and where they know the circumstances in which the offence is to be or is being committed, and where they are aware that there is a real risk that the principal will indeed, commit the offence (see Card, 1995).

Therefore, it is possible that a carer, who allowed a person with HIV and with a learning disability to infect a sexual partner with HIV, might also commit the offence committed by the person with learning disability. This would follow only if it could be said that the carer had the right to stop the sexual activity which does not follow in all cases. It may be the case that the relationship between the carer and the person with learning disability is so much one of dependence and inability on the part of the person with learning disability that the obligation to interfere might arise. Even then, this can only give rise to liability where the carer has sufficient information to realise that there is a real risk, not a fanciful risk, that the person with learning disability might engage in sexual activity. Similarly also, the failure to prevent sexual activity where one (or both) of the parties has a severe learning disability could involve such criminal liability.

It should be remembered that first, criminal liability is only likely to arise where the principal did commit an offence. It should be remembered that the person with learning disability may engage in sexual activity like anyone else, provided he or she has the consent of the other party. It is only when he or she has a severe learning disability within the Sexual Offences legislation that any special liability might arise. Liability does not automatically follow even then. It was decided by the House of Lords Appellate Committee in *Gillick v Wisbech and West Norfolk Area Health Authority* (1985), that doctors would not be guilty of aiding and abetting a man to have unlawful sexual intercourse with a girl under the age of 16 when they prescribed contraceptive

148

treatment to a girl under the age of 16 knowing that she was engaging in a sexual relationship. The best explanation for this decision is, in short, that the doctors would have no choice but to prescribe that treatment. Their choice was either to prescribe the contraception or not. Either way the sex would still take place and the girl, without contraception, would be at risk of greater harm than were the treatment to be prescribed, even without parental knowledge. So also the argument would allow the provision of contraceptive advice and treatment or, it is submitted, sex education to a person with learning disability who had a severe learning disability where the alternative is unsafe sex (in a wider sense than simply the risk of HIV infection). Finally, it should be remembered that a person with learning disability is an adult, not a child under the age of 16, so much greater care should be taken before interfering in that individual's choices.

Obligation of Confidentiality or Freedom to Disclose?
The HIV status of an individual may well be known to the GP of the person concerned. In these circumstances there is a dilemma for the GP, especially if that person's sexual partner is also a patient. Ordinarily speaking, information provided to and gleaned by the GP from a patient is subject to an ethical obligation of confidentiality which may be legally enforceable. However, there are exceptions to the requirement of confidentiality, for example, where a statute requires the information to be passed on. If the patient consents to the disclosure of information, the obligation of confidence of necessity ceases. Such consent may be express or implied, but either way, the patient must be competent to provide the consent which would demand first that he or she understood the commitment to secrecy (see below) and that that commitment was being lost by consenting to the release of information.

Great care needs to be taken to ensure that the patient is indeed competent and also that he or she is not being placed under undue influence to provide consent when the real interests being served are those of the health care providers rather than those of the patient. Of course, this is the justification for disclosure which entitles the GP to apply pressure on the patient by explaining the reasons for wishing to disclose the patient's HIV status to his or her sexual partner or carers. Of course, great care must be taken to ensure that all that is being done is explaining the position and encouraging a decision, whilst making it clear that the person may make whichever decision that they choose, in order that the decision may indeed be regarded as voluntary and not made under undue influence.

149

Amongst the other exceptions to the requirement of confidentiality is the proposition that amongst professionals working in a team, there is a *'need to know'* principle. The essential idea to enable this approach to apply is that the information is to be provided for the use of a team rather than merely the individual to whom it was actually given. If it can be shown that the information is provided to a member of a team for the use of the team, that information can be provided to the other team members when it is necessary so to do. Any other approach would potentially destroy the value of teams such as Community Mental Health or Learning Disability Teams which have to be in a position to share information. Of course, information may in any case be passed where the patient has consented.

There is clearly in law an exception to the obligation of confidentiality when the passage of information is justified by the public interest. However, quite what this means is unclear. What is always required to justify the disclosure is a decision that the public interest in disclosure must be assessed in order to outweigh the private interest in maintaining confidentiality. In *X v Y* (1988), Mr Justice Rose decided the balancing exercise of judicial judgement had to be exercised in favour of preserving the confidentiality of hospital records which would identify actual or potential AIDS sufferers who were doctors. The counter-balancing public interest was the freedom of the press to publish. The balance was exercised in this manner because AIDS sufferers should not be deterred from going to hospital for treatment and the need for a free and informed public debate did not demand the release of the names of the doctors.

Clearly the balance or judgement may be determined differently. Most obviously this might arise where there was someone at serious risk of HIV infection. The public interest might then be thought to justify provision of information to that individual or his or her carers. Indeed the public interest would justify revelation only to those who need to know, therefore in *W v Egdell* (1990) the psychiatrist could reveal his report to the hospital or the tribunal because of the danger he perceived to arise from the patient for whom he had been asked to supply an independent report to a Mental Health Review Tribunal. But this public interest would not have warranted revealing the information to the media. In fact, in some cases it might be the obligation of the doctor to reveal information, as in the American case of *Tarasoff v Regents of the University of California* (1976) where the University was vicariously liable for the negligence of its employees in failing to warn people threatened by a patient who was discharged and killed the threatened person. Kennedy

& Grubb (1994, p.671) conclude that there are such difficulties involved in introducing a *duty to warn* into English law that it is unlikely to occur. However, where the person affected is so obvious as a sexual partner, the courts might take a different view because there is no difficulty at all in identifying the person at risk.

It would seem therefore, that there is some legal justification for the professional guidance to doctors and health care workers when faced with a difficult situation concerning an AIDS patient. The guidance from the General Medical Council (GMC, 1995) commences by identifying the need to make careful judgements about disclosure of confidential information. The first step is for doctors to discuss the implications of the condition, the importance of the security of others and the need to maintain medical care openly and honestly with the patient. It goes on to make clear that a specialist would have to advise the AIDS patient of the importance of informing the GP to ensure continuity of care, and it believes that most patients would easily be convinced of the importance of so informing the GP. If the patient refuses, the GMC identifies two

'sets of obligations to consider: obligations to the patient to maintain confidence, and obligations to other carers whose own health may be put unnecessarily at risk.'

The GMC recommends counselling for the patient about the implications, but if the patient still refuses to authorise disclosure, it recommends that the patient's

'privacy should be respected. The only exception to that general principle arises where the doctor judges that the failure to disclose would put the health of any of the health care team at serious risk.'

As regards informing the patient's spouse or other sexual partner, the GMC

'reached the view that there are grounds for such a disclosure only where there is a serious and identifiable risk to a specific individual who, if not so informed, would be exposed to infection.'

As regards spouse or partner notification, the Department of Health issued guidance in 1992 which identified the benefits of 'partner notification' as being:

'identification of contacts who are given the opportunity to consider whether they wish to be tested; those who have unknowingly been infected may wish to know that they are to enable them to take steps to prevent transmission to others; women who may have been infected may wish to be tested to help them to decide whether to take steps to prevent conception and

151

to help them make decisions about the management of a pregnancy and about breast feeding; access of infected contacts (including children of infected mothers) to treatment and support programmes so that they may benefit from long term monitoring of their clinical condition and from appropriate therapies ... and from appropriate psychological support; identification of uninfected contacts who could also, where appropriate, be counselled about avoiding risky behaviour in the future'

The Department went on to assert that partner notification:

'should be undertaken only with the infected individual's explicit consent obtained without undue pressure'

although the GMCs guidance on exceptions to this rule were noted.

The legal obligation to observe confidentiality may not apply to all people with learning disabilities. As Kennedy & Grubb (1994, pp.640-643) observe, there are two possible approaches to the circumstances under which a legal obligation arises. The first is the 'status' approach, which means that:

'when a child is taken to a doctor for treatment by its parent (and thus becomes the doctor's patient), there arises out of that status relationship a duty of confidence. The implication of this view is that prima facie the doctor has a duty to observe the child's confidences'.

The other, and they argue preferable, view is:

'that the obligation of confidence arises between a child and a doctor when, but only when, the child is competent to form a relationship of confidence, i.e. to understand what secrecy entails. Analytically an approach based upon competence is more in keeping with the general law as regards children since generally the courts, and Parliament, have moved away from a status approach towards a concern for a child's capacity'

Kennedy & Grubb then note that the logic of this approach is that there is:

'no duty of confidence owed to the patient [who has always been incompetent] since the patient is incompetent to enter into a relationship of confidence.'

Whilst noting some particular problems in relation to adults rather than children, Kennedy & Grubb (1994, p.643) affirm the propriety of this approach. It is submitted that it is indeed, the correct approach. Thus there is no restriction on providing information when it is necessary to do so, where the person about whom the information is known is a person who cannot understand what secrecy entails. The downside is that there is then little to stop anyone revealing information as and when they please.

Recognising that this is an *'unsatisfactory state of affairs'*, Kennedy & Grubb suggest that either the courts should be given back the 'parens patriae' power to decide on behalf of adults which was taken away by the Mental Health Act 1959 (a solution which would of course, demand legislation) or the courts should recognise that the doctor/patient relationship is a *'fiduciary relationship from which would flow of course, an obligation not to disclose information when it is not in the patient's best interests to do so'*, (a solution which would simply demand that a court take the appropriate step following, as Kennedy & Grubb point out, the approach of Mr. Justice La Forest in a Canadian case: *McInerney v MacDonald*, 1992).

Compulsory Powers under 'AIDS Legislation'

There are compulsory powers which may be exercised with regard to a person with AIDS. However, they have almost never been used, largely because *'the law is inappropriate to many of the issues raised'* when a person has AIDS (d'Eca & Costello 1995, p.122). The legislation is the Public Health (Control of Disease) Act 1984 under which the Public Health (Infectious Diseases) Regulations 1988 have been made. AIDS is not a notifiable disease, but certain provisions of the 1984 Act (which appear to relate only to notifiable diseases) can be utilised with regard to people with AIDS.

Section 35 empowers a magistrate to order a person to be medically examined where he or she is satisfied, on the written certificate of the public health doctor, *'that there is reason to believe that some person in the district'* has AIDS or is HIV-infected or is suspected of being HIV-infected, *'that in his [or her] own interest, or in the interests of his [or her] family or in the public interest, it is expedient that he [or she] should be medically examined'* and either he or she is not currently receiving treatment from a doctor or the doctor providing treatment consents to the examination. 'Medical examination' includes *'being submitted to bacteriological and radiological tests and similar investigations.'* The magistrate may issue a warrant (under section 61) authorising the doctor to enter the premises.

As d'Eca and Costello (1995, p.123) comment, the *'crucial issue is... the question of interest'*, and they argue that, because there is no cure, *'it is difficult to argue that examination is in the interest of the person concerned or the public'* but that the *'family interest is more problematical.'* Such interest may be present where the sexual partner wishes to avoid infection or where a woman needs to consider the effects of the possibility of infection upon pregnancy and breast feeding. But, even if a medical examination is ordered, there is nothing in the legislation requiring that its outcomes be forwarded to the partner (d'Eca & Costello, 1995, p.123), therefore reliance would have to be placed on whether the obligation of confidentiality applies or if disclosure could be made. Whilst the medical examination may be ordered (subject to penalties for failure to comply), the Act does not deal specifically with the question of the person's consent. A court might decide that the question of consent has been implicitly overruled, although one would normally expect explicit language in a statute to permit this conclusion to be drawn. In any case, doctors are unlikely to proceed without the person's consent (d'Eca & Costello, 1995, p.123).

Section 37 empowers a magistrate to order the removal of a person suffering from AIDS to hospital provided that the magistrate is satisfied that the person's *'circumstances are such that proper precautions to prevent the spread of infection cannot be taken, or that such precautions are not being taken,'* and *'that serious risk of infection is thereby caused to other persons'*, and *'that accommodation for him [or her] is available in a suitable [NHS] hospital'* and that the NHS trust will accept him or her. It is unlikely that this section will ever be used because it is not likely to be an appropriate means of controlling the spread of HIV-infection (d'Eca & Costello, 1995, p.124).

Section 38 empowers a magistrate to order the detention of a person with AIDS as an in-patient in a hospital provided that the person *'would not on leaving the hospital be provided with lodging or accommodation in which proper precautions could be taken to prevent the spread of the disease by him [or her]'* or (as added by the 1988 Regulations) *'proper precautions to prevent the spread of AIDS would not be taken in other places to which the person might be expected to go.'* It is an offence to leave the hospital contrary to the order. Clearly, this section could have very wide application in that it does not simply apply to where the person might live outside hospital but could apply to any place to which he or she might go in the course of daily life. Because of the width of this section, it is possible that it might be used since it could be used to try to prevent a person making contact with other people for sex or drugs. D'Eca & Costello (1995, pp.124-125) report that this section has been applied once in relation to AIDS. They report that the case was dealt with on appeal by consent and so no case law was created. This reflects the fact that the section is not likely to be used and would appear to permit an overly dramatic interference in the freedoms of a person suffering from AIDS.

Section 43 empowers a doctor or officer of the local authority to order that the body of someone who had AIDS and died in hospital *'should not be removed from the hospital, except for the purpose of being taken direct to a mortuary or being forthwith buried or cremated'*, provided that the doctor or officer certifies that in her or his opinion such action is 'desirable'. D'Eca & Costello (1995, p.125) report that this *'section is rarely if ever, used in respect of those who die(s) as a result of HIV disease.'*

Section 44 requires *'every person having the charge or control of premises in which is lying the body of a person who has died while suffering from [a condition associated with AIDS to] take such steps as may be reasonably practicable to prevent persons coming unnecessarily into contact with, or proximity to, the body'*. Sections 43 and 44 may apply so that the body of a person with AIDS who has died may not lie in an open coffin, nor at home (d'Eca & Costello, 1995, p.125).

There is also the AIDS Control Act 1987, which is largely concerned with the collection of data and the reporting of statistics (d'Eca & Costello, 1995, p. 125).

Conclusion
There are a number of problematic legal issues concerning people with HIV infection or AIDS. It has been suggested that most of the law in this area is the same, regardless of whether or not the person has learning disabilities. One of the most obvious dilemmas facing support services and advocates of people with learning disabilities who may be affected directly or indirectly by HIV or AIDS is the balance between the interests of autonomy of the individual and the need to protect others. This is a perennial dilemma facing society in relation to HIV and AIDS. It also faces the learning disability community more widely, not just in relation to the risks of HIV infection, but to sexual expression and the risk of sexual exploitation and to social functioning more widely. When rights and responsibilities come together in the areas of sexuality and HIV, this makes for one of the most difficult balances to strike both morally and legally.

References

Card, R. (1995)   *Card, Cross and Jones: Criminal Law*, Butterworths, London.

Chatterton v Gerson [1981] 1 All England Law Reports 257

d'Eca, C.A.M.E. &   *"Medico-legal aspects of HIV infection and disease"* in Haigh, R.
Costello, T.,   & Harris, D. (1995), AIDS: A Guide to the Law, Routledge, London.

Gillick v Wisbech and West Norfolk AHA [1985] 3 All England Law Reports 402

Gunn, M.J. (1990)   *Consent to Treatment*, 1, The Journal of Forensic Psychiatry 81.

Gunn, M.J. (1994)   *The Meaning of Incapacity*, 2, Medical Law Review 8.

Gunn, M.J. (1995)   *Mental Incapacity - the Law Commission's Report*, 7, Child and Family Law Quarterly 209.

Gunn, M.J. (1996)   *Sex and the Law: A brief guide for staff working with people with learning difficulties*, The Family Planning Association, London.

Kennedy, I. &   *Medical Law: Text with Materials*, Butterworths, London.
Grubb, A. (1994)

McInerney v MacDonald (1992) 93 Dominion Law Reports (4th series) 415

HMSO (1993)   *Mental Health Act Code of Practice*, Department of Health & the Welsh Office, London.

Morgan, D. (1990)   *F v West Berkshire Health Authority*, The Journal of Social Welfare Law 204.
Ormerod, D.C. &   *Criminal Liability for Transmission of HIV*, Web Journal of
Gunn, M.J. (1996)   Current Legal Issues [On the Internet]

R v Clarence (1888) 22, Queen's Bench Division Reports, 23.

R v Mental Health Act Commission, ex parte X (1988) 9, Butterworths Medical Law Reports, 77.

Re C (1993) 149, New Law Journal Law Reports, 1642.

Re F [1990] 2, Law Reports: Appeal Cases, 1.

Roth, P & Gryk, W. *AIDS and Insurance*, in (Eds.) R. Haigh & D. Harris, AIDS: A
(1995)   Guide to the Law, Routledge, London.

Sidaway v Bethlem Hospital Governors [1985] Law Reports: Appeal Cases,
871.

Tarasoff v Regents of the University of California (1976) 131, California Reporter, 14.

W v Egdell [1990] 1, All England Law Reports, 835.

X v Y [1988] 2, All England Law Reports, 648.

Michael Gunn is Professor of Mental Health Law at the School of Law, De
Montford University at Leicester. He has developed a stream of work in
learning disability, particularly in relation to the interpretation of the law
and learning disability and sexuality, and has published widely in this area.

Chapter 11
Policies and Their Contribution to Coherent Decision Making

by Hilary Brown and Paul Cambridge

The aim of this chapter is to outline the contribution which policies can make in the area of HIV and learning disability and also to set out the pitfalls and limitations of written guidance. Policy needs to be enshrined in a number of documents and reflected in day to day practice and management decisions. In this chapter we look at the function of such guidance for developing coherent strategies and setting out how, and by whom, decisions should be made. These statements of intent and structure aim to influence implications for the values and attitudes of staff in services and the opportunities for safer sex education which are made available to service users. Lastly we look at the need for agreed measures for managing HIV risk in services, offering a model set of service principles.

Not Just a Piece of Paper

The term policies is used in the plural as this indicates that we need a many faceted approach. A policy on HIV which is a single document often filed in the bottom drawer of a dusty cabinet, is not going to be enough. A series of inter-locking statements are needed which address process, action and outcomes. These will need to include inter-agency relationships, decision-making mechanisms and other forums for learning and discussion. They will also need to address different audiences and target appropriate guidance to people at different levels in the organisation and the other agencies concerned. The audiences should explicitly span the range of interests in the learning disability community and certainly include users, direct care staff, carers, provider managers, workers in specialist HIV and sexuality services, commissioners and care managers. Some sexuality policies have been developed by explicitly drawing on such a range of interests (Cambridge & McCarthy, 1996).

Later sections of this chapter examine detailed considerations for policy in relation to underlying principles, confidentiality and safer sex education.

159

Specific issues to be covered are likely to include:
1. principles
2. how to use the policy
3. background information on HIV and AIDS
4. housing and support needs
5. confidentiality
6. HIV antibody testing and informed consent
7. assessing and managing risks
8. housing and support rights
9. safer sex education
10. training
11. inter-agency working.

The function of policies should be to structure the way the plans and situations of individual users are approached. They should therefore set the parameters within which staff, both in their individual work and collective discussions make professional judgements and implement shared decisions. In a contentious area, such as sexuality, they also serve to protect individual workers when they make potentially unpopular but principled decisions and to protect the rights of users to sexual expression as well as to protection from exploitation or undue HIV risk.

By creating a structure which establishes general principles *and* sets out how and by whom decisions should be made, the service will effectively own decisions and take shared responsibility for them. This is a vital outcome in any area which demands risk-taking and supportive, rational and coherent management. Individual members of staff would otherwise feel burdened by the weight of decisions or individual service users would be at risk of capricious or inconsistent decisions if each individual member of staff acted according to his or her own values and judgements.

The ideal would be for very specific individual guidance to be given to staff regarding a particular user or circumstance, where responses have been worked out collectively and to the greatest possible extent, in partnership with the user whose life it concerns. Such guidance should clearly reflect the overall philosophy of the service and therefore appear rational to staff, even if they disagree with particular aspects of a decision.

Policies which fail usually attempt to be all things for all people, by trying to anticipate every scenario in which choices might need to be made and setting out detailed prescriptions or instructions for responding. Sometimes situations arise often enough for a generic statement to be useful, for example the first formal guidelines on sexuality published by Hounslow Social Services (1981), made a general 'rule' that if an adult with learning disabilities wanted to be included in a sex education programme and, after consultation, their parents disagreed, then the person's own decision would stand and be supported by the service. A floor to practice was therefore set which would apply in all such cases. Few issues are however, so clear cut or so easily foreseen. The risk with an over-prescriptive policy is that it ties staff into decisions which are overly standardised, blunt and which fail to acknowledge individual needs and circumstances. Similarly, there will be unique cultural aspects and nuances such as religion or ethnicity which need to inform service responses.

Conversely, under-prescriptive policies risk devolving ambiguity and delegating anxiety to those with least power in the system. One staff member interviewed about sexual abuse policies characterised her agency's policy as:

'an uncomfortable fence-sitting exercise, neither addressing the rights of the individual well or fully addressing issues relating to staff protection.' (Brown, Hunt & Stein 1994, p.401).

Such a policy may set lofty ideals but leave people with too much leeway to resolve the issues and conflicting interests in practice. Where there is no *right way*, if policies and procedures are seen or used as a way of covering manager's backs rather than supporting front-line staff, they soon fall into disrepute and disuse.

It is therefore sensible that when individual decisions are the focus of written policy it is more important to set out how to go about making them than to catalogue rules to cover every eventuality. The aim must be to set very clear parameters and channels for communication in order that responsibility is referred upwards as specific guidance and support is passed back down (or across from other agencies). This does not mean that decisions should be taken at a distance from users and direct carers, but that they should be supported and put into practice by those who have the most expertise and resources.

The Function of Policies

Good practice is reflected in individual decisions and planning, the resourcing of relevant options and the development and deployment of staff awareness and expertise. Enabling all staff to tap into a shared pool of information is a vital starting point. Staff may well hold information in different compartments. They may not consider people with learning disabilities to be sexual and hence not sense the risk to them of unsafe sex (Cambridge, 1994). They may be ill-informed about homosexuality or hold homophobic attitudes. They may be unaware of users individual rights in relation to their sexual lives (see Cambridge 1996a). They may not know about the transmission of HIV, the difference between HIV and AIDS or basic information about safer sex (see Cambridge, 1996b). They may not know about local GUM services (special clinics or genito-urinary medicine clinics where people go for advice about or treatment for, sexually transmitted diseases, including HIV counselling and testing). This need for information is particularly acute in relation to sexuality which is still often treated on a laissez-faire basis, as if no intervention from staff would of itself guarantee maximum autonomy for service users. But as the literature demonstrates, without coherent and well planned interventions, people with learning disabilities face their sexual lives with no preparation or support, they risk becoming victims of sexual abuse (see Brown, Stein & Turk, 1995), of having one sided and unpleasurable relationships (see McCarthy, 1994), abusing others (see Charman & Clare, 1992) or having unsafe sex (see Cambridge, 1996c). Therefore the goals of any policies in this area need to include the co-ordination of specialist and generic agencies to create and support opportunities for people to learn about sexual relationships and health in a respectful and explicit way.

A first task, in the new complex web of service agencies which have developed since the introduction of the market in social care, is to identify where expertise currently lies and how it can be accessed. As Paul Cambridge argues in Chapter 1, a bridge needs to be created between specialist HIV agencies and specialist learning disability agencies. Models of joint-work and mutual consultation need to be piloted and developed, as James Nichol has explored in Chapter 3. A balance needs to be maintained between strategic commissioning of service options which require pump-priming and more flexible spot contracts which can be put in place in response to particular needs or situations. Joint commissioning should be explored where a specialist service is likely to be needed by too few users within any one area to be viable or in relation to those services which have both health and social care elements within them.

Accessing specialist advice or services for individuals can be complex and policies should set out at what level such decisions should be taken. Where there are several possible routes into a service, for example, via a GP or a care manager, local guidelines should be developed and collaborative relationships established. Often the critical issue is not only *who pays* but *who knows* about the service and its appropriateness.

Levels of Decision-Making
Good practice in this area involves several distinct elements:
* the creation of a positive sexual culture especially one which redresses discrimination and the frequent *invisibility* of same sex activities and relationships;
* the provision of specialist, explicit sex education and safer sex education for individuals and groups, which is adapted to their needs for information and sensitive to their ways of understanding (particularly important for men with learning disabilities who have sex with men because of the relative lack of such images);
* the capacity to work *with* some individuals to help them to manage risk and on *behalf* of others (such as those who cannot consent or who do not have the capacity to protect themselves) and to protect more vulnerable people from abuse;
* the provision of counselling and HIV testing services to people who may have HIV, which support them emotionally and empower them to access medical services and continue to have safer sex, both for their own and other peoples' health;
* the co-ordination of services to people who have HIV related illnesses, who are ill with AIDS, who need domiciliary or buddy services or who have to receive hospital or hospice based treatment or care.

Mainstream services for people with learning disabilities have tended to address only the first two elements and even then in a patchy way. Although many gay identified men work in sexual health and HIV prevention, including self help and voluntary services and although many bring their experiences of working on HIV and AIDS and their knowledge and commitment into their particular specialisms in the learning disability community, there remains a need for befriending, peer safer sex education and other support links between the learning disability and the gay communities.

Values and Action
Many policies attempt to influence the *culture* of services and to safeguard civil liberties in relation to sexual rights, but the reality is that values are contested within services as much as they are within society at large. Moreover, users themselves may hold conservative views even when these are in conflict with their experiences or behaviours. Heyman and Huckle (1995) document the pervasive disapproval of sex and sexuality by parents and carers which characterises the backgrounds of many people with learning

disabilities and which may well be the source of these attitudes; and Thompson (1994) relates the reluctance of men with learning disabilities to talk about sex with men during sex education.

Moreover there are few consistent ethical frameworks to draw on. Normalisation presents a very muddled view of sexual options (see Brown 1994): men who have sex with men need to challenge and seek to reframe ordinarily *valued options* so as not to adapt to society's devaluation or stereotypical views of their sexuality nor to simply replicate heterosexual norms by wrapping them in a *lesbian* or *gay* cloak.

Different formulations of the principle (see Emerson 1992) place varying emphases on conformity and difference: the North American model argued that people who were already at risk of being devalued because of their disability, should court normalising or status enhancing activities and possessions according to a *conservative corollary*, whereas the Scandinavian model was framed more in terms of rights but within a more segregated context.

The law also provides a contradictory backdrop in that it discriminates against homosexuality between men in relation to the age of consent (18 as opposed to 21) and the provision of what amounts to a private place (the circumstances under which sex is legal), as well as a host of other social and economic irregularities that without general anti-discriminatory legislation, apply to lesbian and gay lifestyles and access to a range of services and resources. It is also at risk of being discriminatory in relation to people with severe learning disabilities who are deemed not to be able to give their consent. The aim of this legislation was to protect people from abuse and exploitation, but it is a blunt instrument when it comes to determining capacity to consent to specific acts within specific circumstances or relationships. Services find the legislation difficult to interpret and to work within, as has been demonstrated by Simon Davies in Chapter 4. The *blanket prohibition* which is effectively established by the law is one which many service workers would challenge, although it provides the only legal protection against abuse or exploitation to some very vulnerable people (see Brown & Turk 1992). A citizenship model would recognise people with learning disabilities as adults with rights which they exercise from a position of multiple inequalities and might include poverty, ethnicity *and* sexuality. But this kind of framework could only work if services develop competence in assessing the functional capacity of individuals to make decisions and take risks. Until services can do this on behalf of individuals there are grave risks in abandoning the safety net provided by current legislation (see also

Michael Gunn's account in Chapter 10).

The extent to which the sexual attitudes of staff towards people with learning disabilities (and specifically towards men with learning difficulties who have sex with men) can be modified through policies is questionable. Rose and Holmes (1991) reported that training was effective to some extent, but Brown, Hunt and Stein (1994) report that within the gendered (and one might also argue by extrapolation *heterosexist*) hierarchies of staff teams, attitudes are more likely to be shaped by real experience than by written guidance. Where staff had passed on concerns to management for these to be dismissed out of hand, they developed a kind of siege mentality which led them to conceal concerns about sexual behaviour and/or to act alone and from personal conviction in seeking to encourage or suppress particular behaviours. It is for this reason that policy development work in sexuality has sought to elicit staff views and experiences at an early stage (see Cambridge & McCarthy, 1996). Positive policy-making needs to be backed up by the explicit sharing of responsibility to assure openness and consistency. Box 1 identifies the main reasons why some policies tend to fail.

BOX I
REASONS SOME POLICIES FAIL

- not disseminated
- too vague or long winded
- contain contradictions between rights and responsibilities
- not backed up with individual planning
- staff lack skills or support
- not implemented with training
- few or no guidelines for practice
- divorce front line staff from managers
- pass the buck to direct care staff
- actual contingencies work against policy
- lack of agreement or ratification
- perpetuate inter-agency confusion
- lost in the new contract culture
- do not reflect the reality of users' experiences and needs
- have no internal co-ordination or focus for responsibility
- do not acknowledge what they cannot achieve
- are not reviewed or updated with experience
- do not help resolve the problems faced by staff

Safer Sex Education

There is an increasing choice of well grounded materials and models of service delivery for sex education and counselling in schools (see David Stewart, Chapter 9), hospital settings (see McCarthy & Thompson, 1992) and specialist counselling services (see Stephen Morris, Chapter 7). Policy and written guidance has the task of ensuring staff know *who* can refer people to these services and *how* to go about it. Moreover many services provide sex education in-house or in the context of self advocacy or other group work. When this is done a proper supervision process should be in place and clear operational boundaries set up with regard to time, place and confidentiality. One obvious area for innovation is to include safer sex education in all such interventions. Where information is offered by care staff within the context of an ordinary caring relationship this should also be discussed in supervision sessions and referenced in individual planning records, as should any sexual behaviour directed towards care staff which is experienced as abusive or inappropriate. We need to remember that such behaviour may be an indication of sexual activity, consenting or non-consenting elsewhere.

Sex educators also need clear guidance about the limits to their role and expertise. They should understand under what circumstances they might need to break confidentiality, for example if a disclosure of abuse, abusing or of high HIV risk behaviour, were offered by an individual in a one to one session or by a group member. They should also be clear about when to refer an individual to more specialist support or assessment (for example to a psychologist). Moreover they should be able to access support and input for themselves, for example through formal supervision or external consultation, such as from a speech therapist who might advise on communication or the choice of appropriate materials or an advisor from a specialist organisation if they need guidance or support about a specific issue, such as challenging sexual behaviour.

Identifying people who need support and/or who are sexually active is a prerequisite for facilitating appropriate access to safer sex education. Staff often assume people with learning disabilities are a-sexual because they do not have the confidence to develop relationships but they also persist in this view even when faced with evidence to the contrary, by minimising or trivialising sexual relationships or even sexually abusive acts when these are witnessed. Men who have sex with men are particularly likely to hide their sexuality or to lack positive role models (Thompson, 1994 & Cambridge, 1996c). In services which have a strong commitment to equal opportunities, lesbian or gay staff will feel able to share their knowledge and awareness of same sex relationships and sexuality to inform positive work with users. In other services they may be silent and invisible.

Who Manages Risk?

By the time an issue becomes framed in terms of risk management it is almost inevitable that decisions should be shared across professional and agency lines. Where individuals are able to benefit from information and support to help them limit risks to themselves or others, that judgement will need to rest on a psychological assessment and be supported by representatives of the purchasing agency responsible for the person's care (such as the care manager or commissioner). Services which fail to *notify* risk, lay themselves open to allegations of negligence in the event that someone *is* harmed. Managed and acknowledged risk is an essential alternative to *post hoc* justifications and excuses: it ensures that ongoing risk can be reassessed and intervention considered again if individuals are unable to protect themselves or continue to behave in ways which poses a risk to others (Simon Davies in Chapter 4 presents a worked example of this kind of power sharing). Action can be taken informally or under Mental Health Legislation if unacceptable risk levels continue from the point of view of an individual's own or another person's behaviour.

People with significant intellectual impairments may not be able to manage high risk situations for themselves, or to consent to participation in sexual activities, medical testing or treatment. A service which fails to note this, hiding behind *empowering* rhetoric allows the reality to allude them. There is nothing empowering about being either out of control or in the grip of other more powerful individuals. The risk manager should draw up a clear contract with the provider agency and through the management line, with direct carers. This should stipulate the degree of supervision or intervention deemed necessary and what signals are to act as a trigger for re-evaluation of the situation and a re-design of the risk management strategy. It is in such situations that advocacy and representation for the individual becomes especially important, as it can help to ensure that any measures taken are in the person's best interests, balanced and regularly reviewed.

Professional judgements may need to take precedence over legal options here and shared planning is the only context within which these can be developed. Supervision or chaperoning of individual men should not take place without clear evidence that it is necessary and a clear rationale as to how it will be implemented. A service instituting such interventions must be prepared to justify it's decision on the grounds that it is in the man's best interest, or in the interests of others (see Brown & Thompson, in press). But what do we need to know to help to take such decisions forward?

Competence in HIV risk assessment is a pre-requisite to informed HIV risk management. Individual rights to sexual activity and opportunities for sexual expression have to be balanced against the risks involved for the person and other people, as much for HIV as for sexual abuse or lower order risks such as crossing the road on the way to the Post Office, which can be equally life threatening. Although people with learning disabilities do not live in a different moral or ethical world, we have a responsibility to acknowledge and respond to their social economic and emotional marginalisation, which makes them particularly vulnerable to these sorts of risk. So far services have developed these skills mainly in relation to recognising and responding to sexual abuse, largely as a result of the work of Brown and colleagues (Brown, Turk & Stein, 1995). For instance, if a man with learning disabilities sexually abuses another person with learning disabilities this is not ignored. Action is taken:

- The abuse is reported according to procedures.
- The reporting officer takes the work forward with staff and managers.
- If necessary an investigation is conducted to establish the nature and extent of abuse and whether other people have been abused.
- The abused person is supported and protected from further abuse.
- People may be notified on a *need to know* basis.
- The abuser may be removed from the service and/or given support concerning his abusive behaviour.
- Staff may be counselled, and so on.

We need the competence to articulate similar responses to managing HIV risk, taking due account of the rights of individuals, the responsibilities of services and the responsibilities of individuals towards others. Service responses will also need to vary according to the nature of HIV risk. The responses to managing HIV risk for men with learning disabilities who have unsafe sex in public toilets (Cambridge, 1996c), varied from keeping people at home or supervising people when out (and in one case included an HIV test for the person) to assertiveness work and HIV counselling. The former would clearly reduce HIV risk by restricting high risk behaviours or limiting opportunities, but would also directly affect the right to sexual expression and opportunities to meet people, move independently and interact in the wider community.

Services therefore need to decide on appropriate responses when they discover someone they support is putting themselves at risk of HIV. But it will be almost impossible to assess what level of risk is reasonable by extrapolating from our own personal responses, as people approach risk assessment and risk management very differently at an individual level. Priorities depend on the various circumstances, demands and preferences in their lives, as there are complex costs and benefits to sex and sexual encounters and the assessment of associated risks. What services *can* do however, is ask some basic questions about peoples' understanding and appreciation of sex, safer sex and risk.

- do they know they are putting themselves at risk of HIV (that they can get HIV from sex)?
- do they know they can still have sex and reduce their risk of HIV (safer sexual alternatives to penetrative anal or vaginal sex)?
- do they know about safer sex (when and how to use condoms during penetrative sex)?

If the answer to any of these questions is no, then the service clearly needs to intervene to provide additional education and support. Moreover, if there are wider disincentives to practicing safer sex (such as access to condoms or pressure from a partner), more complex service responses are likely to be required. Without such a basic assessment the service cannot assume that the user is making an informed choice about having unsafe sex. There are further questions that can be used to help fine tune service responses to risk management. These include:

- do they understand what HIV is and how it is easily transmitted through unprotected anal or vaginal sex?
- do they know that they *can get* HIV from unprotected anal or vaginal sex, whether they are penetrating or being penetrated?
- do they know that they *can give* HIV to someone from unprotected anal or vaginal sex, whether they are penetrating or being penetrated?
- do they know that HIV leads to AIDS and that AIDS is an illness that people die from?

If the answers to one or more of these questions is yes, then this may mean that the person is acting irresponsibly in the knowledge of risk as well as some of the possible ways to respond to reduce risk. But as we have heard from Stephen Morris in Chapter 7, the explanations for risk behaviours may be deep and complex and work may be needed with individuals on a number of fronts and this work may need to be sustained for long periods of time. We have seen similar messages from Michelle McCarthy and David Thompson (Chapters 6 and 5) that a long term approach is similarly desirable for sex education. But services have a duty of care and that sometimes means protection if the person is unaware or unconcerned about the risks involved. An argument could be constructed that short term measures should be taken to restrict or eliminate the behaviours that lead to high HIV risk. If someone was going out on their own and getting beaten up, the service would seek to stop this happening, but like other risks such as smoking, the nature and consequences of the risk are sometimes perceived differently, in that they are seen not to demand an immediate response.

A service which knowingly allowed someone to cause physical or sexual harm to another person would be failing in its duty of care. The same principle has to apply to HIV risk and harm. Although the management difficulties and resource consequences of responding to HIV risk need to be acknowledged to help to remove disincentives to recognition, the much stronger rationale for responding on both moral and legal grounds (as Michael Gunn has demonstrated in Chapter 10) has to be firmly embedded in policy, hence the imperative to respond to HIV risk and to determine the nature of the person's risk-taking and an appropriate response or intervention.

In an ideal world people would respond to knowledge about whether they might have HIV and how they can avoid giving it to someone else if they do have it. This knowledge would need to be based on a reasonable understanding of the nature of their own risk and risk behaviours, both past and present and the potential consequences of unsafe sex for themselves or others. They would also need to demonstrate an understanding of AIDS, illness and death and the links between unsafe sex and HIV transmission. This is a complex chain of inter-connections and possibilities, and can be more simply approached by asking:

- is the contact mutual or exploitative? If it is exploitative, then there is a clear case for intervening to stop it, regardless of HIV risk.
- is the behaviour high risk? If they are having unprotected anal or vaginal sex then there is clearly a significant risk to be managed, whereas oral sex or other sexual contact could be assessed as low risk and requiring a lower priority intervention.
- does the person at risk know about safer sex and is she or he physically able to practise it? If not, then they should receive intensive safer sex

education, have access to condoms and receive ongoing staff support and monitoring.

- Is the person at risk able to insist on safer sex and that they or their partner(s) use condoms for high HIV risk activities such as penetrative anal or vaginal sex. If not, they should receive counselling and education for negotiating skills, assertiveness and HIV.

This relies on services taking steps to minimise HIV risk to the individuals they support and having the ability to demonstrate through intervention and programmes that they have taken reasonable steps to educate people to risk, assess informed consent, provide appropriate supports and minimise opportunities for exploitation. The equation is also about peoples' rights, however, and people should be enabled to express their sexuality and practice the sex they like in rewarding ways whenever this does not conflict with service responsibilities to protect people from undue risk. Safety should be assured whenever possible through safer sex education and HIV counselling, rather than policing sexuality or restricting consenting and mutual sexual activities (see case study below).

Principles for Policy

We have identified ten key principles which we believe should underpin and inform policy in HIV in learning disability services and which can be used to help map the more detailed content of policies. These are presented below in the form of statements of principle, followed by a brief exploration of the implications for practice.

1. Services have a responsibility to promote the sexual health of service users. This means providing information about HIV and AIDS, safer sex education and support and advice in practising safer sex and/or reducing high HIV risk behaviours. Staff and service users should have access to appropriate safer sex education resources and use them as identified and laid out in the policy. Service users who are sexually active, at risk of HIV infection or worried about HIV or AIDS have a right to safer sex education and information about the transmission of HIV.

2. Services and staff have a responsibility to assess and manage the risk of HIV infection in relation to individual service users. This means that staff should have broad skills in recognising and assessing risk of HIV infection and be able to respond and manage risk in appropriate ways to protect vulnerable users from unacceptable risk. Specialist staff should

171

have the knowledge and competence to practice this principle. Service users have a right to support in reducing their risk of HIV infection and in helping them to manage risk, without compromising their rights to sexual expression. Service responses to HIV risk should, wherever possible, be empowering rather than controlling.

3.   **Services and staff should not discriminate against service users on the basis of their known or suspected HIV status**. This means that there should be non-discriminatory policies and practices in relation to HIV, the provision of services, and other resources (such as staff support) for service users. For instance, no service user should be excluded from appropriate services or have staff support withdrawn on account of their HIV status. Service users have a right to appropriate and equivalent services and support regardless of their HIV status or of the unfounded opinions of staff about people with HIV or the risk of HIV transmission.

4.   **Staff should not be discriminated against on the basis of their known or suspected HIV status**. This means that there should be non-discriminatory employment practices and staff support. Employees should not have to put up with inequitable treatment or disadvantage in relation to their known or suspected HIV status and have the right to be treated equally and fairly. They should not be subject to insult or abuse, whether from other staff or service users and should have access to management support and counselling services.

5.   **People receiving services are entitled to confidentiality and support in relation to their HIV status**. This means that service users who disclose their HIV positive status to managers or staff should have this treated confidentially. Staff should only be informed of the HIV status of service users on a need to know basis according to criteria laid down in the policy. Users who are HIV positive have the right to respect and dignity, including privacy and confidentiality. They are also entitled to receive counselling in relation to their HIV status.

6.   **People employed by services are entitled to confidentiality and support in relation to their HIV status**. This means staff who disclose their HIV positive status to colleagues or managers should have this treated confidentially and under no circumstances should such information be disclosed to service users. Staff who are HIV positive have the right to respect and dignity, including privacy and confidentiality. They are also entitled to receive counselling and specialist support in relation to their HIV status.

7.   People supported by services should be discouraged from seeking an HIV test unless informed consent can be independently validated. This means that staff and managers should not persuade or encourage a service user to have an HIV antibody test unless they are satisfied that the individual is prepared for this and both able and willing to consent. Informed consent should be assessed independently of the service and people have a right to full information about the advantages and disadvantages of HIV testing, including the possible consequences and implications of testing positive.

8.   Service users should be informed of their rights in relation to sexuality and HIV and also their responsibilities in relation to safer sex. This means that service users should have straightforward information in the form of words and pictures which explain their rights directly or as part of a programme introduced by staff which conveys their rights and responsibilities. These include the right to have safer sex and the responsibility to practice safer sex.

9.   Staff should be informed of the policies and their implications for practice and supported to implement relevant guidance. This means staff should receive training to understand the implications of policy statements, setting out service values and how these can be achieved. They should have a basic knowledge of HIV and AIDS and its implications for people with learning disabilities. Staff have a right to access information and support from managers in relation to how HIV and AIDS impinges on their work and practice.

10.   There should be a named service contact competent at providing advice and support and implementing policy. This means a key service contact or outside practitioner available to all staff who is able to explain policy and offer advice about interpretation. This would include risk assessment, risk management, confidentiality and guidance about what to do in specific situations. They would have the competence and knowledge to respond in line with the agency's policy and its aims and procedures.

Addressing Confidentiality

Every person has a right to privacy and respect about their lifestyles and sexuality including people with learning disabilities supported by community based services (McCarthy & Cambridge, 1996). Written guidance on sexuality should outline the details and reasons for this. Not everyone chooses to talk about their sexual lives with others. Some people only tell close or trusted friends who they know will be able to help them with difficulties or advise them what to do if they have worries or concerns. Others feel comfortable telling lots of people about their sex and relationships. Some people would prefer not to be told things about someone else's sexuality. It is therefore not easy to establish any hard or fast rules about this.

People with learning disabilities are no different. Sometimes service users ask staff about their private lives or about the sex they have. Staff may not feel comfortable disclosing such information or may judge it inappropriate to tell someone else. Alternatively they might feel able to respond in an open and appropriate way, feeling that the question was a natural thing to ask and that their closeness with the person as a keyworker or support worker warranted an honest response. Conversely when staff are in the position of seeking information they also need to acknowledge boundaries. Answering a question or concern a service user may have may mean asking additional questions to clarify things. If someone is embarrassed, then this should be obvious and a useful point for drawing the line of privacy. Although information shared between two individuals should be regarded as confidential unless there are clear reasons to the contrary, when one person is a service worker and the other a service user, the former has a duty to share relevant information with managers in order to ensure that a consistent approach is formulated. Information belongs to the agency rather than to individual members of staff and should be noted properly in records to ensure continuity when staff leave or their responsibilities change. The detail and type of information recorded should be subject to scrutiny, with due regard to confidentiality and access.

If someone discloses an abusive incident or unsafe sex during ordinary conversation or sex education, this will have potential implications for service responsibilities and may need to be taken further. For example, a male user discloses unsafe sex in public toilets or a woman service user sexual abuse by a member of staff or a more able service user. It is in such situations that rights and responsibilities conflict and decisions have to be made in relation to confidentiality. It is also in such situations that the support and guidance of co-ordinators in the service should be sought, not necessarily by disclosing names or breaking confidentiality. Whatever happens, the person's views should be sought and the situation explained to them.

This may not necessarily be such a dilemma as many suppose, because the keyworker or sex educator should anyway have agreed the *rules* with the person before starting the work. There is also a big difference between telling a colleague and telling someone in the service who is also aware of the importance of confidentiality and guidelines for handling sensitive situations.

Considerations of confidentiality are particularly important in relation to sexuality and HIV, because some people have been verbally and physically abused or discriminated against on the basis of their suspected or known HIV status, or simply because of their sexuality. Not all men who have sex with men are gay identified. Some are in heterosexual relationships and identify as straight and we know that many men with learning disabilities have sex with men and that very few identify as gay (Thompson, 1994). It is therefore important that considerations about confidentiality in relation to HIV are also linked with confidentiality in relation to sexuality. This discussion can be condensed to four key points in relation to confidentiality and HIV:

1. Service users who are thought to be practising unsafe sex, sex with people from high risk groups, or other HIV risk behaviours such as injecting drug use with shared needles or dirty works (drug injecting equipment) are entitled to confidentiality.

2. Service users who have expressed a wish to take an HIV antibody test and/or for whom informed consent has been assessed as valid are also entitled to confidentiality.

3. Service users who are tested for HIV, whether the result is negative or positive, are entitled to confidentiality in relation to the test and its result.

4. Service users who have HIV or AIDS and are under the supervision of their GP or consultant at a GUM clinic for monitoring or regular check ups, are entitled to confidentiality in relation to their HIV status or related illnesses.

Staff with such information or concerns should approach the key service contact without disclosing their concerns to other people. It may be decided that there are good reasons to inform other staff, for example in situations where

• someone working with the sexual partner of a person who is suspected or found to be HIV positive would need this information to help with risk assessment, risk management or providing safer sex education to them or their partner;

• a designated support worker might need to help a service user who is HIV positive with their diet, medical check ups or attending outpatient clinics;

175

- it would be the job of a service manager, care manager or broker to help secure appropriate services for the person and to co-ordinate appropriate social and health care inputs.

Similarly, a service user's suspected or known HIV status should not be disclosed to another service user, as there are other ways of addressing issues of risk, protection and support. The responsibility for making these decisions and deciding on *need to know* lie with the HIV co-ordinator who should be an experienced senior practitioner and/or manager. In some cases, the HIV co-ordinator may need to consult with service managers or outside specialists/consultants.

Training Needs

There is a wide choice of sex-education and staff training resources available for addressing sexuality and HIV issues in learning disability. Training managers are usually responsible for developing training programmes and purchasing training for provider organisations and this needs to be matched to the policy, competence of staff and changing needs of service users. As with training initiatives on sexual abuse at agency and inter-agency levels (Stein & Brown, 1995) evaluation of such interventions can identify effectiveness but also any gaps in implementation. In HIV, the specialist competencies of managers and the HIV co-ordinator will need to be met, in addition to the general staff training needed to develop mainstream competence and to help implement and maintain the effectiveness of policy. Induction training for new staff should similarly reference HIV. It is often the case that staff simply need basic information and reassurance about HIV and AIDS which challenges some of the myths associated with infection and transmission (see Cambridge, 1996b).

Support staff and keyworkers who are interested in, and competent at, working on sexuality and HIV should be available to provide ongoing support and reinforce the messages from formal education, although policies will need to acknowledge that no person within the service should be expected to provide advice and support on sexuality or HIV if they do not have the motivation, or find the subject difficult or embarrassing. There are also likely to be religious or cultural reasons why some people will not wish to become involved in this activity.

The education of service users about sexuality, HIV and AIDS is an important component of policies and underpins implementation by fostering empowerment. A wide range of sex education and safer sex education resources are available, including booklets, teaching packs, drawings and other written or pictorial materials. There is also a selection of videos, mainly designed for groupwork and sex education groups. Such resources vary in coverage, detail, key messages, social context, role models, attention to equal opportunities and the values which drive them. It is therefore important to agree on a range of resources to use for specific purposes which are in line with the principles and philosophies of the service. Some HIV and safer sex educational materials fail to represent homosexuality or safer sex in accurate ways, marginalising sex between men, despite this being a priority for HIV prevention. Those resources for sex and safer sex education considered most appropriate in terms of their usability, effectiveness and suitability should be referenced in policies and made available for training and education.

There are five key aims in relation to providing sex and safer sex education which policies and guidelines will need to address.

1. Safer sex education should be provided as an integral part of all sex education programmes designed at the individual or group levels.
2. Sex and safer sex education should be provided to all service users as part of an ongoing programme of education and support for sexuality and HIV.
3. Specialist sex and safer sex educators should be responsible for designing, delivering and reviewing the HIV elements of the programme, whether specially trained key educators from within the service or specialist educators from outside.
4. Sex and safer sex education should be provided in accordance with individual programmes agreed as part of the individual planning systems in response to assessed needs.
5. Staff involved in delivering sex and safer sex education should receive supervision and support from managers.

Case studies provide a useful device for trainers and managers who wish to examine the robustness of a policy or the competence of staff to navigate what amount to complex moral dilemmas and conflicting rights and responsibilities at the individual and service levels. It is also important to acknowledge that decisions are sometimes made on the basis of only partial information and that service responses will often need to be flexible and adapt to changing circumstances or knowledge, viz.

• *A young man with learning disabilities is known to cottage regularly in a local park. He discloses to his keyworker that he often has receptive oral and anal sex with different men but rarely do those men use condoms. The service response would initially aim to reduce the risk of HIV infection by safer sex education and counselling about HIV risk and transmission. Condoms would be made available or he would be helped to buy them. He would demonstrate his intention to use them and the reasons for this, and there would be an attempt to monitor his success in practising safer sex. If this did not work then there would need to be more intensive therapeutic or psychological interventions. At some point the other risks of his behaviour, such as the legal situation and risk of getting beaten up would also need to be explained. Intervention would also need to explore issues of sexual identity, self image and so on and alternative opportunities to express his sexuality or socialise identified and discussed.*

• *It is subsequently found that this man occasionally has sex with an older man with learning disabilities in the service whom he penetrates anally. If this was found to be consenting on the part of the other man and if the other man could confirm extra strong condoms were used and was aware of the importance and reasons for practising safer sex and if the sex was in an appropriate place then there would be no need to intervene. If it was found to be exploitative of the older man then there is clearly a case to intervene to stop it. If the younger man refused to use condoms and the older man was unaware of the risk, then there would be a case to intervene to provide intensive safer sex education and support for the older man and counselling for the younger man about his responsibilities to practice safer sex.*

• *It is also subsequently disclosed that this man has regular vaginal sex with a young woman with learning disabilities. She considers him to be her boyfriend and has had minimal sex education and does not know about HIV or safer sex. She wants the relationship to continue. He considers the relationship to be casual. There would need to be intensive counselling work with the man on issues relating to his responsibilities to practice safer sex and on personal and emotional relationships. His responsibility towards others for HIV and emotional risks would need to be addressed. The young woman would need intensive individual work on safer sex and contraception and ongoing support in relation to her emotions and feelings. She should be helped to become more assertive and independent of him and make informed decisions about continuing the relationship based on the*

178

*different risks involved for her. She should demonstrate her intentions
and ability to insist on protected vaginal sex.*

New Partnerships

Services for people who are HIV positive, and/or have become ill with HIV
related illnesses or AIDS, need to be provided in partnership with other specialist
agencies with the aim of *bridging* rather that duplicating skills. Sexual
health is acknowledged as a priority within the Health of the Nation strategy
(1995), but work will be needed to ensure that mainstream services do not
marginalise people with learning disabilities in meeting their wider targets
or aims. Complex negotiations already take place in relation to health and
social care needs and responsibilities and these will need to be adapted to
reflect the involvement of various health and social services input to people
with learning disabilities. Simpson (1994) recently reviewed access to sexual
counselling services and did not find them equipped or committed to offering
services to people with learning disabilities. Disability awareness may need
to be built into their contracts and supported by training and appropriate
consultation.

It is clear that if people with learning disabilities who are at risk of HIV, and
more specifically men with learning disabilities who have sex with other
men, are to have appropriate access to preventative education, support,
treatment options and health services, prejudices must be dispelled. Explicit
policies can provide a framework for good practice: safeguarding the civil liberties
of users and setting up channels through which staff can access information,
professional expertise and appropriate services. Policies fail when they try to
stipulate *what* rather than *how* decisions are to be made. But they also fail
if they are not clearly enshrined in contracts, job specifications and quality
standards, or if the pressures of the work in new devolved and deregulated
service structures militate against the sharing of responsibility. When that
happens people with learning disabilities who are at risk from HIV are likely
to get too little help too late. They should be helped to get the best advice,
support and services, and to get them in time.

References

Brown, H. (1994)   *An ordinary sexual life?: A review of the normalisation principle as it applies to the sexual options of people with learning disabilities,* Disability and Society, 9(2), 123-144.

Brown, H., Hunt, N., & Stein, J. (1994)   *Alarming but very necessary: Working with staff groups around the sexual abuse of adults with learning disabilities,* Journal of Intellectual Disability Research, 38, 393-412.

Brown, H., Stein, J. & Turk, V. (1995)   *Report of a second two year incidence survey on the reported sexual abuse of adults with learning disabilities,* 1991 and 1992, Mental Handicap Research, 8(1)1-22.

Brown, H. & Thompson, D. (in press)   *A minefield in a vacuum: the ethics of working with men with learning disabilities who have unacceptable or abusive sexual behaviours,* Disability and Society.

Brown, H. & Turk, V. (1992)   *Defining sexual abuse as it affects adults with learning disabilities,* Mental Handicap, 20(2), 44-55.

Charman, T. & Clare, I. (1992)   *Education about the laws and social rules relating to sexual behaviour,* Mental Handicap, 20, 74-80.

Cambridge, P. (1994)   *A Practice and Policy Agenda for HIV and Learning Difficulties* British Journal of Learning Disabilities, Vol.22, No.4.

Cambridge, P. (1996a)   *The Sexuality and Sexual Rights of People with Learning Disabilities: Considerations for Staff and Carers,* BILD, Kidderminster.

Cambridge, P. (1996b)   *HIV and AIDS and People with Learning Disabilities: Guidelines for Staff and Carers,* BILD, Kidderminster.

Cambridge, P. (1996c)   *Men with learning disabilities who have sex with men in public places: mapping the needs of services and users in South East London,* Journal of Intellectual Disability Research, Vol.40(3), June.

Cambridge, P. & McCarthy, M. (1996)   *Developing and implementing sexuality policy for a learning disability provider service,* Health and Social Care in the Community,

Emerson, E. (1992)   *What is normalisation,* in (Eds.) H. Brown & H. Smith, Normalisation: A Reader for the Nineties, Routledge, London.

Health of the Nation (1995)   *A Strategy for People with Learning Disabilities,* Department of Health, London.

Heyman, B. &   *Sexuality as a Perceived Hazard in the Lives of Adults with*

Huckle, S .(1995)   *Learning Difficulties*, Vol.10, No.2, p.139-157.

Hounslow Social   *Guidelines on Personal Relationships, Sexuality and Mentally*
Services (1981)   *Handicapped People*, Hounslow Social Services Department,
                  London.

McCarthy, M. (1994) *Against All Odds: HIV and Safer Sex Education for Women with
                  Learning Difficulties*, in (Eds.), L. Doyal, J. Naidoo & T.
                  Wilton, AIDS: Setting a Feminist Agenda, Taylor and Francis,
                  London

McCarthy, M. &   *Your Rights about Sex: a Booklet for People with Learning*
Cambridge, P.   *Disabilities*, BILD, Kidderminster
(1996)   .

McCarthy, M. &   *Sex and the 3 Rs: Rights, responsibilities and Risks*, Pavilion,
Thompson, D. (199)Brighton.

Rose, J. &   *Changing staff attitudes to the sexuality of people with mental*
Holmes, S. (1991) *handicaps: an evaluative comparison of one and three day work
                  shops*, Mental Handicap Research, Vol.4, No.1, pp.67-80.

Simpson, D. (1994) *Sexual Abuse and People with Learning Difficulties: Developing
                  Access to Community Services*, Family Planning Association,
                  London.

Stein, J. &   *All in this together: an evaluation of joint training on the abuse*
Brown, H. (1995) *of adults with learning disabilities*, Health and Social Care in
                  the Community, Vol.3, No.4.

Thompson, D.   *Sexual experience and sexual identity for men with learning*
(1994)   *disabilities who have sex with men*, Changes, Vol.12, No.4.

Hilary Brown is Professor of Social Work and Community Care at the Open University. Prior to her appointment she was senior lecturer in learning disability at the Tizard Centre, University of Kent at Canterbury, where she directed a programme of research and consultancy on sexual, and other, abuse of vulnerable adults, including joint input to the first nationally funded incidence study of reported sexual abuse of adults with learning disabilities.

Index

Self image v, 12, 23, 178
Semen 12, 13, 18, 19, 31
Sex education iii, v, vi, vii, 2, 3, 4, 5, 7, 9, 10, 11, 12, 13, 14, 18, 19, 20, 21, 22, 23, 24, 25, 28, 46, 49, 50, 57, 59, 62, 71, 72, 82, 84, 85, 87, 88, 89, 92, 95, 96, 98, 99, 100, 101, 102, 117, 125, 126, 127, 129, 131, 134, 135, 136, 137, 147, 149, 159, 160, 161, 163, 164, 166, 171, 174, 175, 176, 177, 178, 181
Sexual abuse vii, 6, 9, 23, 24, 28, 49, 50, 53, 58, 77, 82, 96, 99, 111, 113, 124, 129, 132, 161, 162, 168, 174, 176, 180, 181
Sexually transmitted diseases 31, 50, 81, 90, 162
Staff training 5, 10, 13, 20, 22, 23, 28, 54, 55, 57, 59, 67, 69, 134, 137,
Testing (HIV) vi, 7, 9, 14, 15, 16, 22, 34, 80, 122, 139, 163, 173
Therapy 39, 97, 102, 103
Transmission 31, 41, 78, 170, 171
Treatment (HIV/AIDS) v; 10, 14, 17, 29, 31, 37, 38, 39, 41, 43, 102, 104, 105, 106, 107, 140, 141, 149, 150, 152, 153, 156, 162, 163, 167, 179
Unsafe sex 4, 18, 20, 23, 65, 74, 79, 82, 83, 119, 149, 161, 162, 168, 169, 170, 174, 175
Vaginal sex 11, 18, 133, 169, 171, 179
Videos 120, 177
Virology (HIV) v, 14
Vulnerability vii, 5, 65, 66, 90, 130

185

Other books published by bild in this field:

Sexual Health Education for Children and Young People with Learning Disabilities: A Way of Working
by Karen Adcock and Gill Stanley 1996
(published in collaboration with Barnados)
ISBN 1 873791 38 0 - £15.00

HIV and AIDS and people with Learning Disabilities
by Paul Cambridge 1996 a series of three booklets:
What you need to know about HIV and AIDS
ISBN 1 873791 61 5 - £3.50
a guide for parents
ISBN 1 873791 66 6 - £2.50
a guide for staff and carers
ISBN 1 873791 71 3 - £3.00
Series ISBN 1 873791 76 3 - £7.50 the set

Your Rights about Sex
by Michelle McCarthy and Paul Cambridge 1996
ISBN 1 873791 52 6 - £5.00

The Sexuality and Sexual Rights of People with Learning Disabilities: Considerations for Staff and Carers
by Paul Cambridge 1996
ISBN 1 873791 73 9 - £5.00

Personal Relationships and Sexuality: Policy Statement and Guidelines 1992
(report published in collaboration with the West Midlands Learning Disability Forum) - £3.50

For a full listing of all bild books and for further information about our other services, write to
BILD,
Wolverhampton Road,
Kidderminster DY10 3PP
or telephone 01562 850251